THE HIDDEN DESIGN OF HUMANITY

Breaking the Code of Da Vinci

DANIEL WALTERS

THE HIDDEN DESIGN OF HUMANITY

FIRST SUNBURY PRESS EDITION
Printed in the United States of America
September 2012

ISBN 978-1-620061-04-6

Published by:
Sunbury Press
Mechanicsburg, PA
www.sunburypress.com

SUNBURY PRESS
Mechanicsburg, Pennsylvania USA

Table of Contents

Introduction.....................................1
.

Proportions of Humanity...................2

Vitruvian Man Drawing...................12

My Da Vinci Man............................39

The Design of the Body...................78

The Original Design......................100

Bibliography.................................110

Introduction

This man; drawn to fit so well within a circle and a square, is one of the most well known drawings in the world. It's another masterpiece by Leonardo da Vinci. The name of the drawing may elude your memory; but if you were to see him, you would know him. He is The Vitruvian Man; so named by da Vinci for the Roman architect Vitruvius, who first described him in a book about architecture. Many artists have tried to draw this man of what Vitruvius described, but it was da Vinci who made it into a masterpiece.

There is still so very little known about how da Vinci created this drawing. The information; gathered from his drawings, have been found on the unfinished notes he jotted down here and there. His work was intense, but scattered; leaving us with an extremely hard task of trying to think like da Vinci.

How would he have approached the problem? He probably first entertained the idea from reading the books written by Vitruvius; but he didn't use this description as a strict template, he also went a few steps further with the drawing. This kind of initiative lets us know that he put a lot thought into the drawing. He didn't merely sit down one day and draw it; he would have investigated the problem first. I could see him watching passers by; studying how they move, and how their body is proportioned, comparing them to everybody else passing by. He may have noticed that each individual's arms are proportioned the same; whether your short or tall, it didn't seem to matter. He would have seen how different each one of us could be; but he would have also seen how we all could be alike in so many ways.

Da Vinci would have tested what Vitruvius wrote; and would have tried to push the boundaries of how to place the body within the circle and the square. He would have made measurements of the different positions; recorded those measurements with a sketch, and then made several more sketches to double check his work. After exhausting every possible defining calculation; da Vinci would have seen a design hidden away; evolving throughout human history.

It's a common ratio of how our body is designed, and the basic form our bodies must adhere to. It has taken many twists and turns on its journey through humankind, and still this one design would have to have an Adam and Eve starting point, a place that was as close to this ideal form as we can find. With the help of learning about how and why the Vitruvian Man drawing is so important.

It would be da Vinci that would take what Vitruvius had wrote about in his books, and make the perfect Vitruvian Man. This drawing is the key to unlocking the one basic model that is in every human being from Adam and Eve up to modern day. The best way to unlock this intricate design of nature; is by exploring the Vitruvian Man drawing in a more comprehensive way, and trying to understand it in the same manner that da Vinci may have. We will describe the units of measure that are found within this design, and the best way to use those units to design the body of what the earliest modern human being may have looked like.

Proportions of Humanity

Throughout history, it has been proposed that there should be a way to predict the ideal proportions of the human body. It began with the ancient Greeks, but I believe it was a Roman architect by the name of Marcos Vitruvius Pollio that finally started to understand the true proportions of the human body.

"Vitruvius is the author of *De architectura,* known today as *The Ten Books on Architecture,* a treatise written of Latin and Greek on architecture, dedicated to the emperor Augustus." [3] Within these ten books on architecture, he describes a way in which it would be possible to measure with a standard of measurements. The example he uses is the human body, because it was believed that the human body had within itself a perfect set of proportions. In his Book 3, Chapter 1:1; *On Symmetry: In Temples and in the Human Body,* he says, "Without symmetry and proportion there can be no principles in the design of any temple, that is, if there is no precise relation between its members, as in the case of those of a well shaped man." [4] I believe he was trying to say that all buildings should have a perfect proportion in order for those buildings to be solid, useful, and beautiful. He seemed to have noticed how a well balanced structure would last over time and still remain in good working condition if it's constructed with a balanced proportion to all its intricate parts, like a human body.

He describes his ideal man in Book 3:1:2 as, "For the human body is so designed by nature that the face, from the chin to the top of the forehead and the lowest roots of the hair, is a tenth part of the whole height; the open hand from the wrist to the tip of the middle finger is just the same, the head from the chin to the crown is an eighth, and with the neck and shoulder from the top of the breast to the lowest roots of the hair is a sixth; from the middle of the breast to the summit of the crown is a fourth. If we take the height of the face itself, the distance from the bottom of the chin to the underside of the nostrils to a line between the eyebrows is the same, from there to the lowest roots of the hair is also a third, comprising the forehead. The length of the foot is one sixth of the height of the body, of the forearm, one fourth; and the breadth of the breast is also one fourth. The other members too, have their own symmetrical proportions, and it was by employing them that the famous painters and sculptors of antiquity attained to great and endless renown." [4]

He then describes a way in which the human body relates to a circle and a square in Book 3:1:3. He says, "Similarly, in the members of a temple there ought to be the greatest harmony in the symmetrical relations of the different parts to the general magnitude of the whole. Then again, in the human body the central point is naturally the navel. For if a man be placed flat on his back, with his hands and feet extended, and a pair of compasses centered at his navel, the fingers and toes of his two hands and feet will touch the circumference of a circle described there from. And just as the human body yields a circular outline, so too a square figure may be found from it. For if we measure the distance from the soles of the feet to the top of the head, and then apply that measure to the outstretched arms, the breadth will be found to be the same as the height, as in the case of plane surfaces which are perfectly square." [4]

His description of the human body was a first for his time in around 50 – 150 B.C. "This work is the only surviving major book on architecture from classical antiquity." [3] It seemed to have disappeared until the mid – 1400's. This is probably when it fell into the hands of Leonardo da Vinci.

"The illegitimate son of a 25-year-old notary, Ser Piero, and a peasant girl, Caterina, Leonardo was born on April 15, 1452, in Vinci, Italy, just outside Florence." [5] Florence is where he was probably exposed to the writings of Vitruvius as an apprentice to Andrea del Verrochio. "From 1485 to 1490, Leonardo produced a study on loads of subjects, including nature, flying machines, geometry, mechanics, municipal construction, canals and architecture (designing everything from churches to fortresses). Also during this period, Leonardo produced his first anatomical studies." [5]

Da Vinci's work is astounding; and he pioneered research in how the human anatomy is structured and how it works. He had piles of notebooks with his research and he made many discoveries. Some people believe him to be the first biometric engineer, but one thing has always been clear to me.... He was an artist. He was an excellent artist that studied the human body, not unlike many of the artist of today.

Leonardo da Vinci created his depiction of what Vitruvius described in those architectural books around 1487. This drawing, named after Vitruvius, became one of his most famous drawings. He was the first to create a drawing that more accurately depicts what Vitruvius envisaged that the ideal man should be. "This image exemplifies the blend of art and science during the Renaissance and provides the perfect example of Leonardo's keen interest in proportion." [6]

He would have made several different sketches of the Vitruvian Man; and then he would have recorded the measurements he made on those drawings. If he did make several other drawings, where are they? Could there be more drawings like the Vitruvian Man, by da Vinci, out there somewhere? I would love to see how his drawings would look as compared to my own. That's one of the biggest things I keep wondering, if he was really exploring the proportions of a human body, then why didn't he draw more than the one and only drawing of the Vitruvian Man? Who knows?

I'm going to break down da Vinci's own words on the drawing to show how da Vinci inadvertently began to show the world a hidden design of how the human body functions as a "structure of nature". He tried for such a long time to better understand how it works by doing something that was unheard of in his time. He studied cadavers; he moved them into different positions to find out how the many different joints worked, he took measurements of every movement, and then he described what he discovered with his drawing, the Vitruvian Man. I believe that this drawing is one of his greatest creations, because with it we can lay the foundation to every person's proportions walking on earth. One problem, however, he used mainly cadavers, and rigor mortis would have set in. That means when he made some of his measurements, the body wouldn't have reacted in the same manner as a living body. It wouldn't have been as flexible; therefore some of his assumptions could have been wrong. If he did make some of those adjustments; they were never described by his hand; those notes haven't been found yet.

The idea of a universal set of proportions for the human body has been explored since ancient times. Thus far nobody has discovered this golden mean of proportion for the body, but if you look around at all the different people and watch closely where their hands touch, just below the waist while standing, you will notice that just about everybody's hands are placed in about the same location. Why is that? Could it be that we all have basically the same proportion? Well, in fact we do all share about the same DNA. "Almost all (99.9%) nucleotide bases are the same in all people." [1] You see it's the 0.1% that makes us different than anybody else. The human body is predictable in the fact that we know the body should have a certain amount of parts, like one heart or two legs, and those parts should also have an average size. If these parts are missing or they don't work correctly, then we expect that there is something wrong with that body. The reason we expect this is because we are naturally accustomed to seeing the average human body with every new person we see, but if we see someone or something out of that normal, then we naturally assume there's something wrong.

That 0.1% of DNA is what will give us our individualism; it will tell our body how tall we'll be, what color of hair, and all the other little details that make us who we are. That's the stuff that makes us who we are and it gives us that distinctive look we crave so much.

The genes we carry will also be influenced by its environment that it's "carried" through. That's why even identical twins will have a slight difference in their DNA. The environment is what your body is put through, physically, mentally, and chemically. A lack in nutrients will do damage to your body, so therefore it will influence your DNA. Mutation of genes can also lead to a difference in your body's proportions, like a mutation in a gene that involves the growth factor. It will tend to lead to a difference in the proportions in the long bones as compared to the rest of the body.

This could be looked at in how cells are formed. If they are formed incorrectly, then wouldn't they be out of proportion to the rest of the body or the part it has helped form? If it was a machine with working parts, and one part is not correctly proportioned, then the whole machine won't work correctly either. Each cell carries information about how to proportion itself as one individual part of the whole part; and if that information in that one individual cell is wrong, then it would affect the part as a whole, therefore that part would either not work correctly or not fit properly as it should according to the information carried by genes. For example, if a body is born with an enlarged heart, the mutation will cause the body to have problems working properly. This could cause shortness in breath, dizziness, lack of oxygen to the brain, and many other problems.

I believe that we all have a destined proportion for our body, because as humans, we all tend to look and work in the same manner. Where could this information about our proportion lay, I don't know for sure, but I believe that within that 99.9% of DNA that we all share; there's a proportional marker that tells our body what we should look like in a general form, and then the 0.1% that we hold dearly as individuals, tells our body how we should look with our own personality. The proportions of that body would stay the same, no matter how tall we are or how large our body is, we still remain at that same basic proportion. Even when there's a mutation of those genes, our body will still tend to remain at the proportion as governed by the normal and also by mutation.

For example, a person with achondroplasia will tend to stay the same proportions governed to it by its mutated genes. "Dwarfism is a result of autosomal dominant mutation in the fibroblast growth factor receptor gene 3 (FGFR3), which causes as abnormality of cartilage formation. FGFR3 normally has a negative regulatory effect on bone growth. In achondroplasia, the mutated form of the receptor is constitutively active and this leads to severely shortened bones." [2] The body will then receive the alternative form of proportions, and then it will stay at this form for the rest of its life.

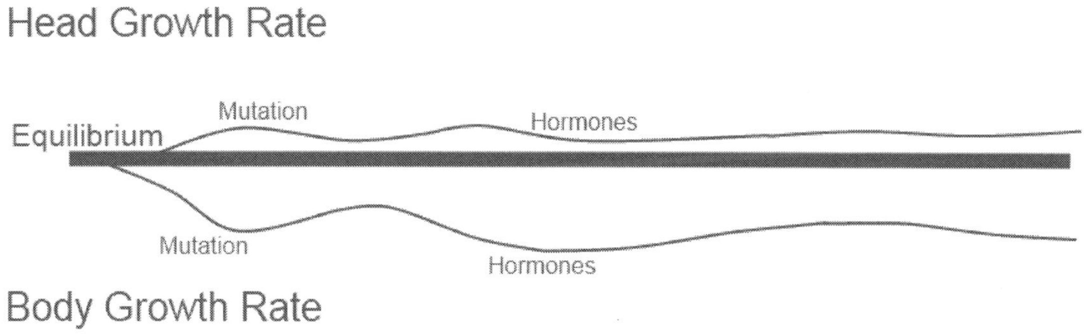

Figure 1

As our body grows; there will be many different factors that will steer our body away from the equilibrium, like a small mutation, or even something as simple as hormones. These factors may pull our body away from that equilibrium; but we still tend to stay as close to that general form as possible. That's what makes us who we are; if not, then how could we describe what a human body generally looks like.

If we were to take three Sycamore seeds right off a mature tree; plant them during the spring, and watch them grow for a few years, would they all grow into identical trees? Of course not; they would all be different in some way. One tree may have had to battle with a larger tree for sunlight; and grow with a crook in its top branches. One may have been planted in some sorry soil; therefore making it hard to retain any nutrition, and causing its growth to be stunted. The other may have been placed in the perfect spot, and received all the attention it needed, growing into a beautiful large tree.

All the trees first started out in what would seem to be the same size, color, and shape seed; but they all ended up different. They would have the same information inside that little seed to tell it to grow tall and strong like the other Sycamores; but it was their environment that would ultimately shape how those little trees would turn out.

They are different as individuals, but the same as a whole. To define the general form of the Sycamore tree is to define the general form of an average tree: roots, trunk, branches, and leaves; but to define it as an individual Sycamore tree, we would describe each part of the general form of tree with greater detail. For example: the roots grow more branch like in shallow soil, the trunk is white underneath the molting bark and has a knot four feet from the ground with part of a fence growing out from the middle, the branches are spread out to shape a beautiful oblong cloud, and the light green leaves are broad and full of life. So while the plants all start with the same size and shape as a seed; they will all grow into an individualized plant but still retain the same proportions as the other plants of the same kind. We as humans will start from one cell and then we will grow into our own individualized form, all the while retaining the same proportions governed to us starting at that one cell. At birth the skull is not fully developed and some of the roof plates are still not fused together. “The bones of the roof of the skull are initially separated by regions of dense connective tissue called “fontanels”. There are six fontanels: one anterior (or frontal), one posterior (or occipital), two sphenoid (or anterolateral), and two mastoid (or posterolateral). At birth these regions are fibrous and movable, necessary for birth and later growth.” [8] As growth continues, the fontanels are replaced by sutures. “The posterior fontanel usually closes by eight weeks, but the anterior fontanel can remain open up to eighteen months.” [8] After birth the body is approximately a 1:4 ratio, the head is larger than the rest of the body.

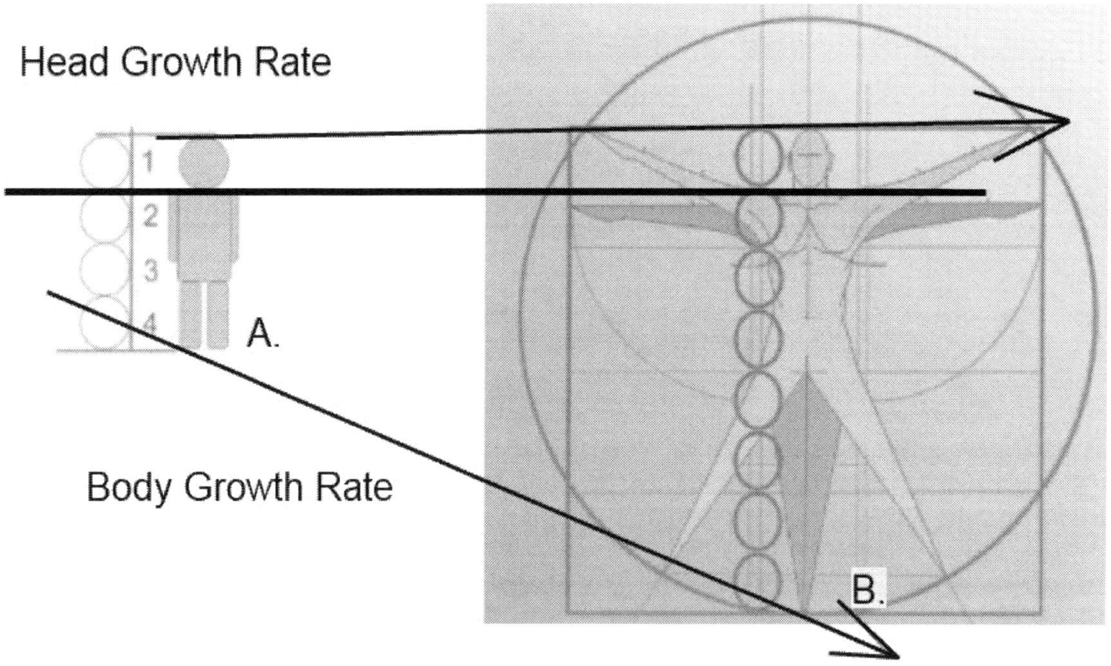

Figure 2

The first three to four years of human growth are extremely rapid; at this time, I believe the body is trying to reach its predetermined body design. In Figure 2, point A., at birth our bodies are measured; with the measurement of the head length as a benchmark, four heads tall, on average. “Height and weight show rapid growth in infancy and puberty and show ‘S-type’ growth patterns, whereas brain, head circumference, and visual organs are of the neural type and grow up to 80% of the adult size by age 4.” [9] The head at this time is foreshortened, because the... “growth of the mandible was primarily in a horizontal direction for the first 3 ½ years of life and that in some cases the glenoid fossa moves posterior as much as 10mm during this time." [10] Studies have shown how the mandible grows horizontally in the first 3 ½ years rapidly and then it slows in growth, but still grows throughout our life until we reach adulthood. At this time, as it seems, the head is not at the proportional size until about 3 to 4 years of age, but then when it all reaches its proportional design, it seems to stay there, unless the DNA or growth hormones are interrupted by something in our environment.

This one idea of how our body changes its proportions is a hard idea to swallow; but there's a lot of information about how this change takes place. The body doesn't look like it; but there is a significant change right after birth; but it's so common we tend to overlook this major detail in the way our body changes.

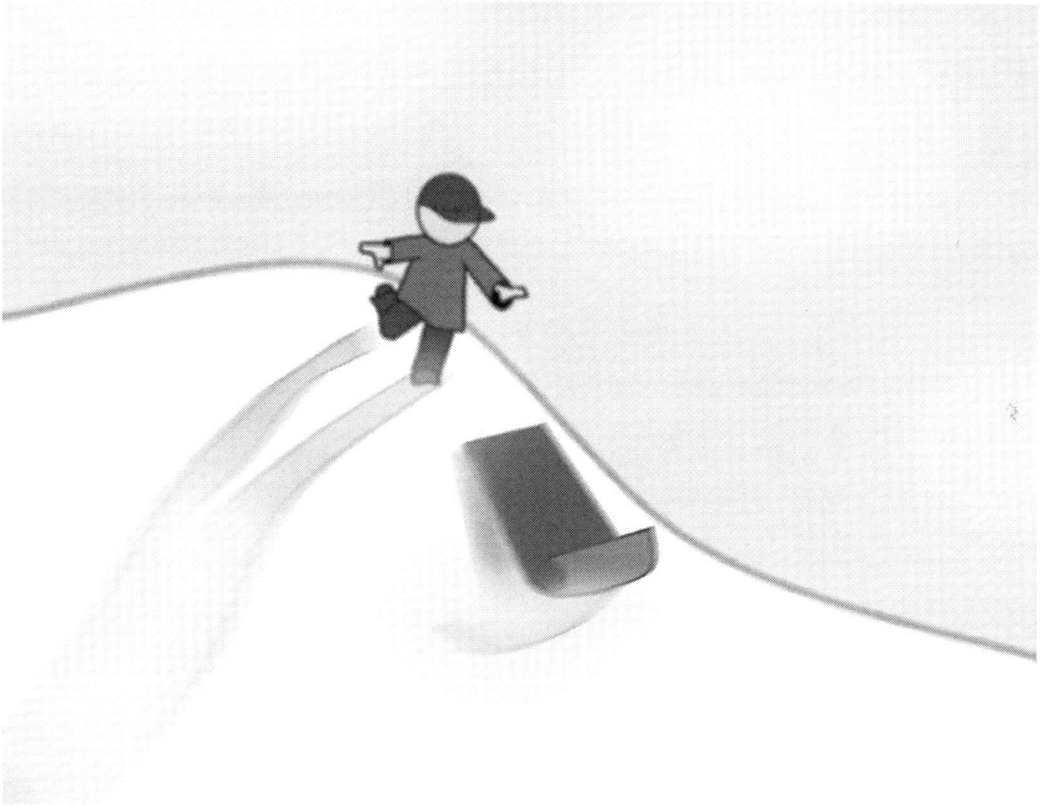

Figure 3

The best way I can think of to explain how this works is by looking at Figure 3; the sled represents the growth of the head, and the boy represents the growth of the rest of the body. They both start at the same point; the top of the hill, but let's say the sled (the growth of the head) gets an early start, and is rushing down the hill without the boy (the growth of the body). This would be the beginning of growth of the fetus; head first. In order for the boy to catch up; he will have to run faster than the sled, but once he does catch up to the sled, they both will slide down the hill at the same rate.

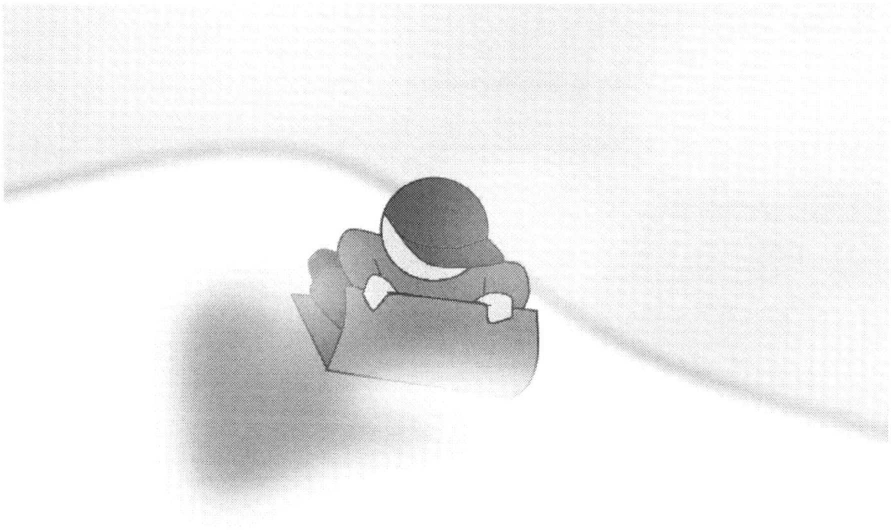

Figure 4

This would be the same way the head growth catches up with the body growth; as soon as they both reach the same rate (Figure 4); they tend to stay at this same rate the rest of our lives.

As our mandible grows horizontally, our torso and appendages will also grow at this same rapid growth rate. When we reach this 1:8 ratio; we can see how our appendages work more proficiently at this certain ratio. The body will then gain its new found balance, and it will begin to work as a more intricate machine of nature. As the body develops, we also figure out the best ways to use our body. When we are little, we stumble around trying to figure out how to better use our body; like learning how to walk, talk, and eat. The more we did any of these, the more we learned how to better use our body in order to accomplish our goals.

In Figures 5 and 6 (next page), we can see a steady growth from about age 3 years old up until adulthood. With such a steady growth, we can see that it conforms to a linear equation. If this is correct, shouldn't we be able to find this linear equation? Since the body grows at a rapid rate at different stages of growth, this linear equation would be difficult to find. You would have to consider each stage of growth in this equation, but each body grows at a different rate. So if it's not possible to find this equation of growth, then how can we assume that we can predict the proportions of that body as it grows?

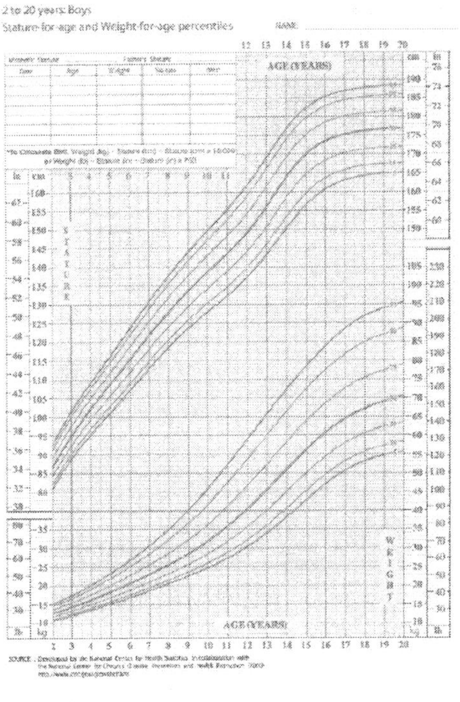

Figure 5

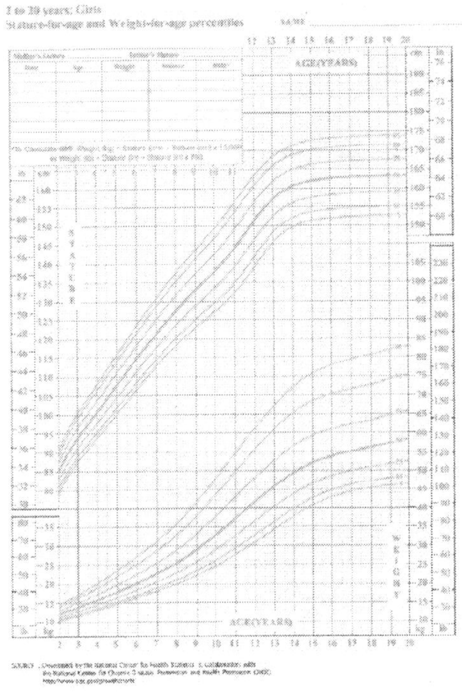

Figure 6

When we talk about proportions; we shouldn't only think that it's how each part is sized as compared to the rest, we also need to remember that it's also having the right amount of parts for each body when it's formed at the beginning of life. This equilibrium that most of us begin with as a general form of a body; one head, two eyes, two arms, and so on, has made it easier for us to survive. Our genes would only want to keep those proportions that would help the body to better perform and that would help it survive.

Let me discuss what proportions really are and how it forms the body as a whole part. "1.part of whole: a quantity of something that is part of the whole amount or number. 2. Relationship between quantities: the relationship between two or more amounts or numbers, or between the parts of a whole. 3. Relative size: the correct or desirable relationship of size, quantity, or degree between two or more things or parts of something." [12] No matter how tall or how fast we grow, our body will remain proportioned the same throughout our life. So even through those growth spurts our body will try to remain at its own balanced design.

The recent research into DNA may have not been around for da Vinci to investigate; but I think he still would have seen this pattern, he would have picked upon the idea of a more intricate design, far more thought out than any other drawing of the Vitruvian Man. He may have not known about DNA; but he still could have seen how closely we all look alike. His extensive notes about the human anatomy tell us that he was exceedingly passionate about the proportions of the body. His painstaking works in finding this form probably began with several other sketches, notes about his measurements, and maybe even his reasoning on why he placed the body in both the circle and the square. In order for us to fully understand why it was so important to da Vinci; I believe we need to try to think more like da Vinci.

We need to understand how the final drawing was made; what other drawings could be made with the same concept in mind, and if they all relate to one another. There could be a common thread between the different sketches. This would be a great way to really crawl around in da Vinci's head; to show the work that he may have done in order to prove to himself that we do have a common form.

Those secrets inside that genius mind would forever be locked away; if we were to never find the other notes, how could we truly know how this drawing was really supposed to be used. The Vitruvian Man is the final drawing of a culmination of several other drawings; we could assume it was meant to be used as a key. This would be used to measure the general form for anyone with this same common ratio.

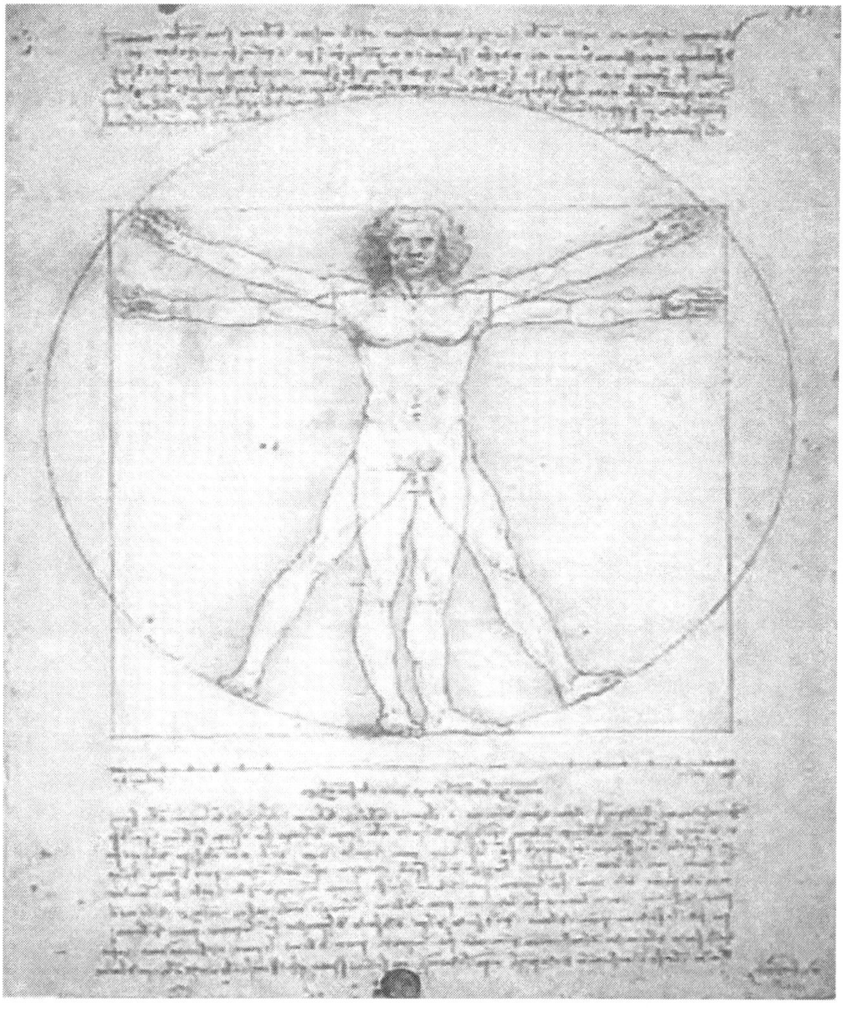

Da Vinci also wrote at the bottom of the drawing, "From the roots to the bottom of the chin is the top of his head is one eighth of his height; from the top of the breast to the top of his head will be one sixth of a man. From the top of the breast to the roots of the hair will be the seventh part of the whole man. From the nipples to the top of the head will be the fourth part of a man. The greatest width of the shoulders contains in itself the fourth part of the man. From the elbow to the tip of the hand will be the fourth part of a man; and from the elbow to the angle of the armpit will be the eighth part of the man. The whole hand will be the tenth part of the man. The foot is the seventh part of the man. From the sole of the foot to below the knee to the beginning of the genitals will be the fourth part of the man. The distance from the bottom of the chin to the nose and from the roots of the hair to the eyebrows is, in each case the same, and like the ear, a third of the face." [7]

These writings would be his conclusion to his own research into the proportions of a human body. It gives us only a little bit of information on what he believes is the common form for all of us. He shows no proof to the design anywhere on or around the drawing. He leaves that up to us to find out.

We will need to do a little reverse engineering; beginning with the drawing. It'll be done step by step; trying to stay within what clues that da Vinci wrote down around the drawing.

Vitruvian Man Drawing

My Vitruvian Man is based on the drawing made by da Vinci, described by da Vinci and Vitruvius, but with my own touch. Let's begin by looking at what da Vinci wrote down at the top of the drawing, "Vitruvius, the architect, says in his work on architecture that the measurements of the human body are distributed by Nature as follows: that is that 4 fingers make 1 palm and 4 palms make 1 foot, 6 palms make 1 cubit; 4 cubits make a man's height. And 4 cubits make one pace and 24 palms make a man; and these measures he used in his building."[7] This is a description of how he measured the Vitruvian Man; it's a key to how we should measure the drawing, and he put this key on the drawing. He put it just below the drawing; a straight line with a few small marks. Look at Figure 1A.

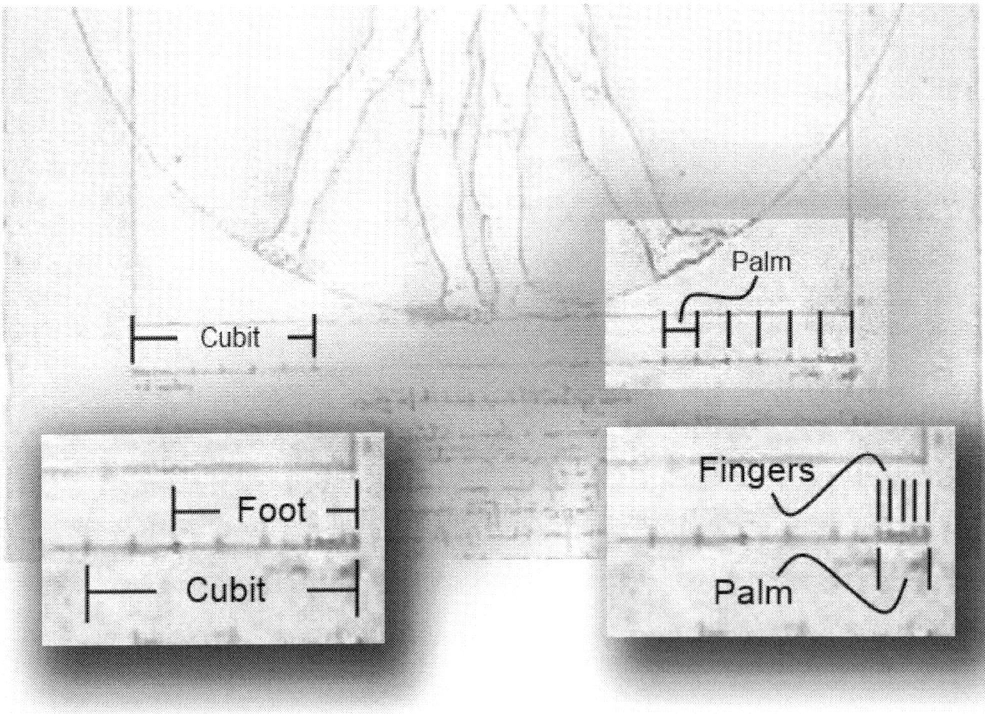

Figure 1A

In Figure 1A, we can see how the key works; it his measurement of the cubit broken down by what Vitruvius wrote in his book, but scaled down for a smaller drawing. He shows us that 4 fingers make 1 palm and 6 palms make 1 cubit. Now let's make a grid that will be 4 cubits tall; to make a man's height.

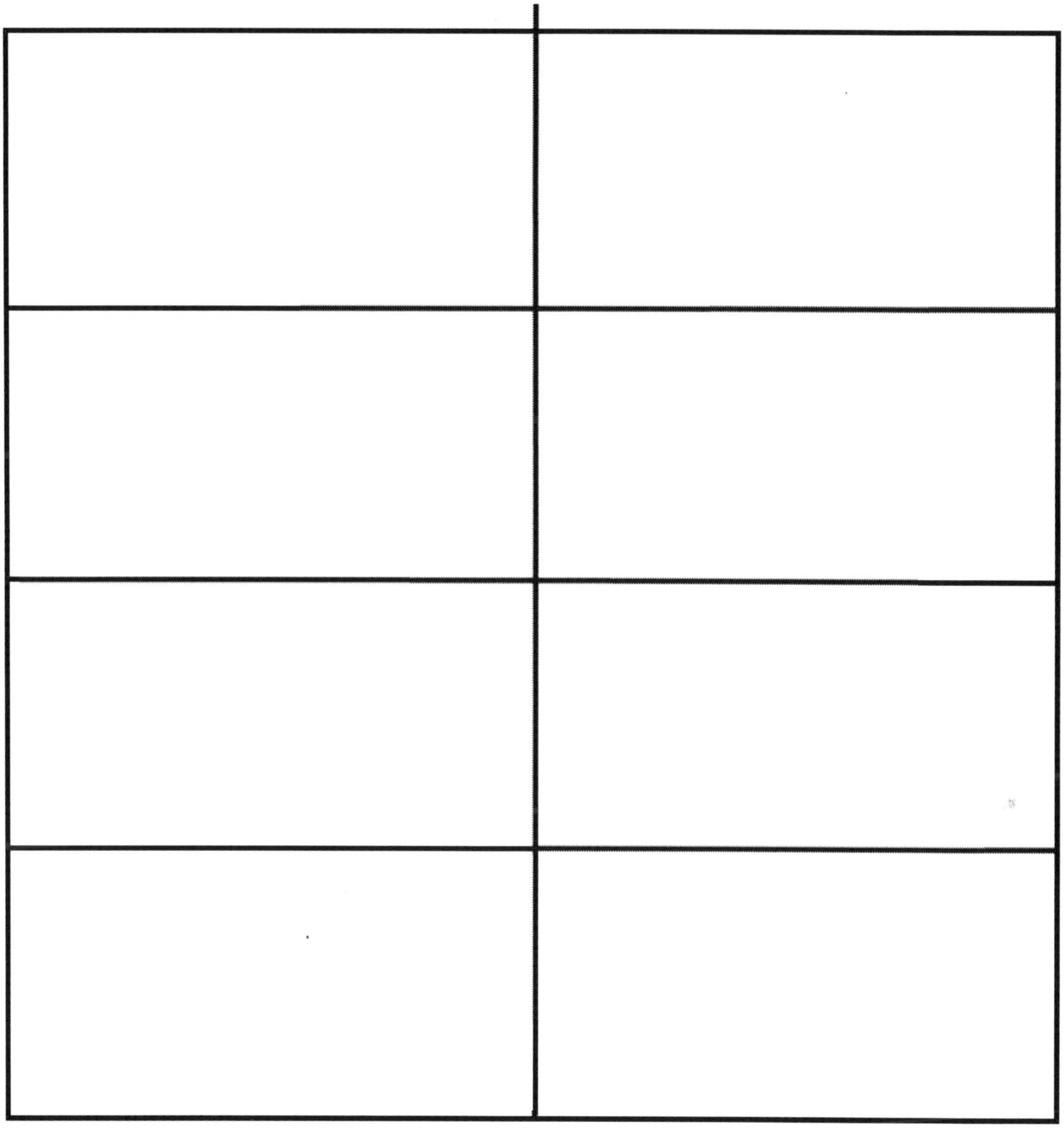

Figure 2A

Divide the square in Figure 2A in half vertically; and then into four equal parts horizontally. The square should look like the one in Figure 2A. This will make it the desired 4 cubits. To better see how these cubits could form a body; let's place a grid over the Vitruvian Man drawing, as seen in Figure 3A.

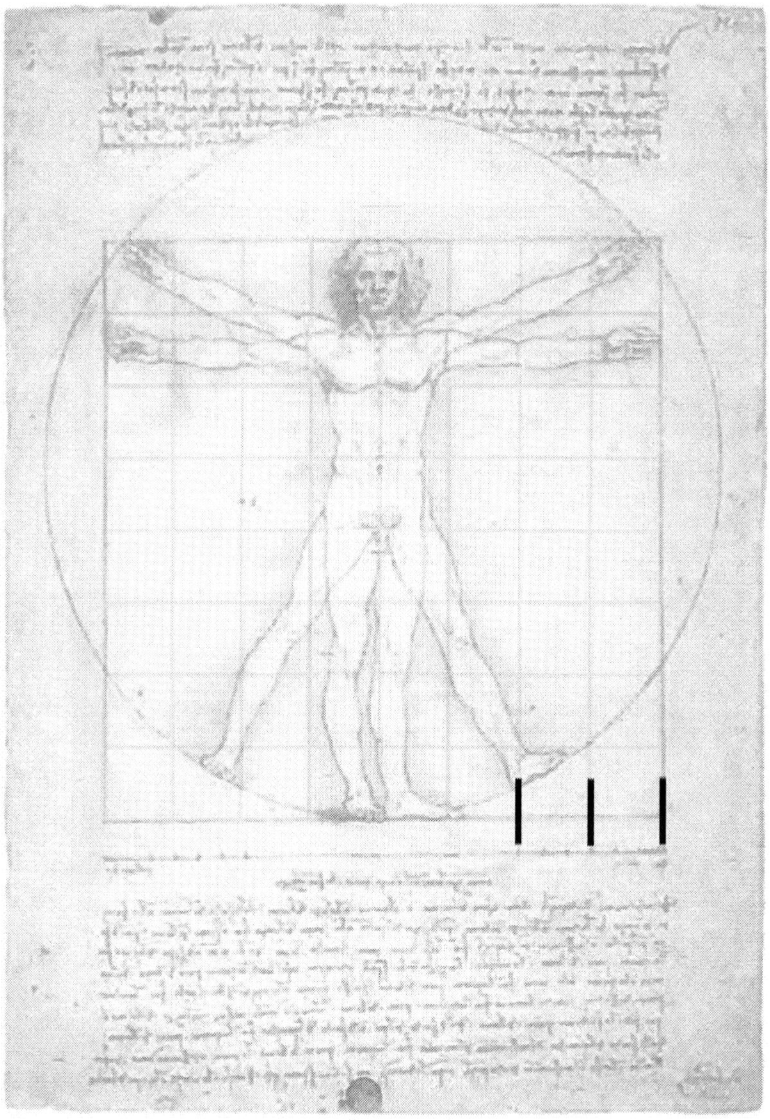

Figure 3A

Can you see the measurement key just under the drawing? Notice how the grid is formed by squares that are ¼ the size of a square cubit. To draw a head that's 1/8 the size of the square in length; it should be the same length as one of the grid squares; and for the width of the head, it should be approximately 5/8 the size of the head in length. For a 5 inch square the head should be 0.625 inches in length and 0.390625 inches in width. It should be centered on the vertical center line at the top of the square, as seen in Figure 3A.

Draw two lines that measure ¼ of the square's length apart; draw those lines vertically also, centered with the center line; as you can see this would be the length of one cubit. For a 5 inch square the ¼ Lines will measure 1.25 inches apart. Draw two lines that measure 1/5 of the square's length apart; draw those lines vertically, centered with the center line. For a 5 inch square the 1/5 Lines will measure 1 inch apart.

Measure down from the top of the square a distance that's 1/6 the total length of the square; draw that line horizontally, as seen in Figure 5A. For a 5 inch square the 1/6 Line will measure approximately 0.8333 inches from the top of the square. When making these measurements, it is necessary to take into account the width of the pencil lines in order for it to be more accurate. With such a small drawing that width could cause your drawing to be less accurate.

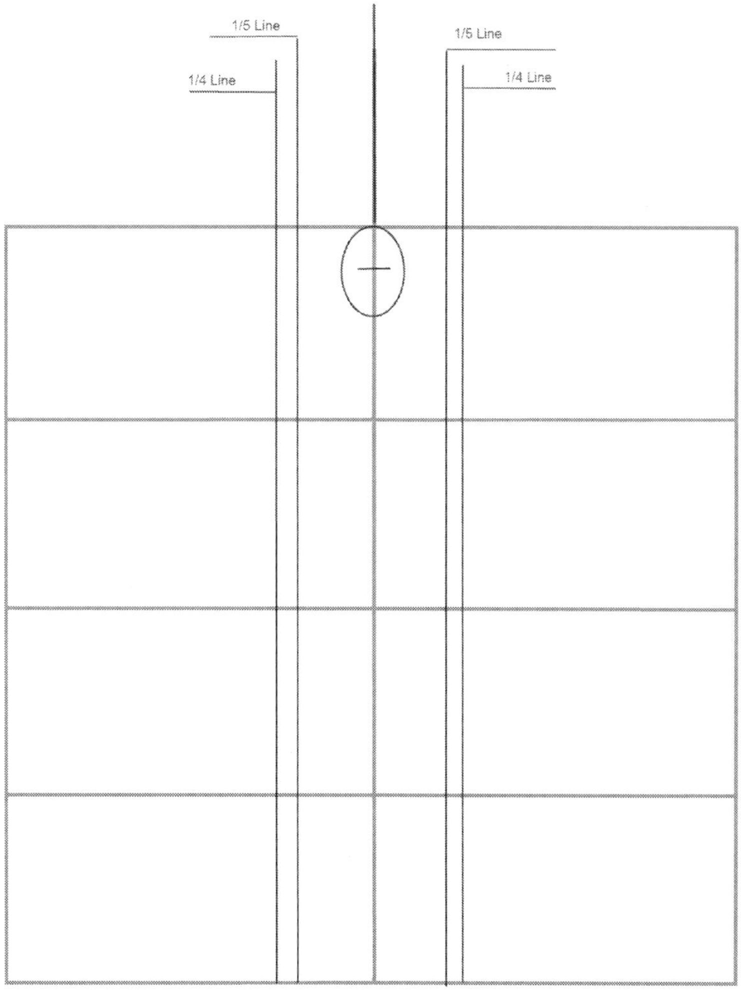

Figure 4A

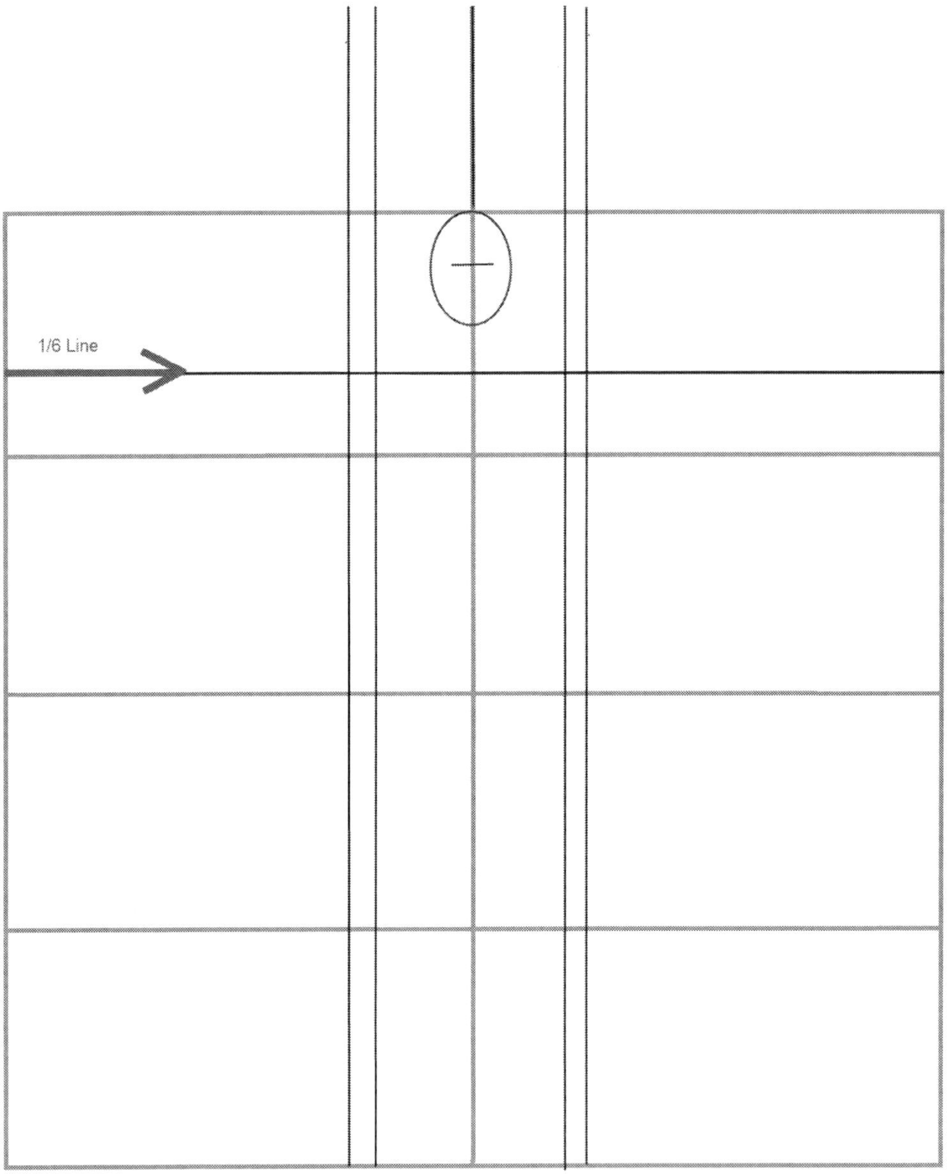

Figure 5A

Draw a body with the arms outstretched and the legs to the center. The arms should be drawn along the 1/6 Line out to the edge of the square. My human body is more of a stylized form of a body, because I want to be able to follow what da Vinci has in his notes and on his drawings without getting confused. I want to be able to see what he saw without having to strain to look past all the details of finely drawn body. Most artists are taught to begin with this simple form; it's a kind of building block that we have to build upon in order to better proportion each body that we draw.

So leave out any unnecessary details, like fingers, eyes, mouth, and even the feet for now. Right now the most important thing we are trying to do is to draw the basic form at first; before we can make it into an individual. The proportions should always come first; and measuring those proportions will be easier to measure with just a basic form to begin with. It's easier to move the body around, make any slight adjustments, and to correct any mistakes, without having to redraw a complete picture.

This body doesn't represent what a perfect human body should be; it merely provides us with the foundation. There are very few people that would have a body that looks the exact same as our drawing; so don't get hung up on the finer details, and concentrate on only the proportions. This way you can see where everything should be more accurately and the rest of the details of the individual body can be drawn later.

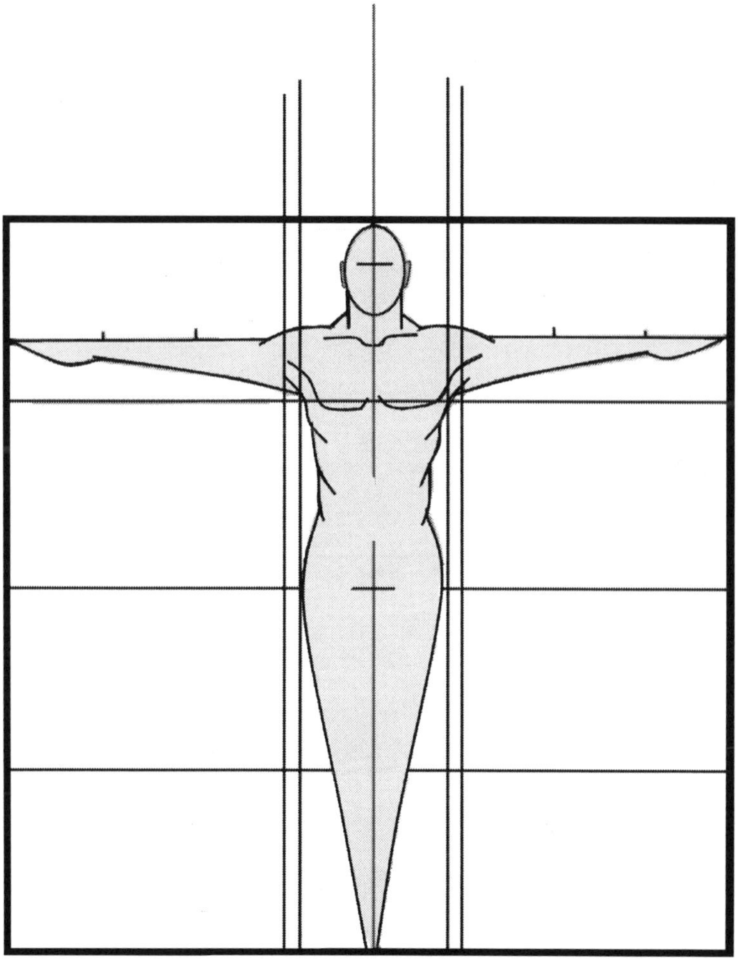

Figure 6A

Now, this is where da Vinci's drawing is so different than anybody else's drawing. His new and inventive idea is as he says, "If you open your legs so much as to decrease your height 1/14 and spread and raise your arms till your middle fingers touch the level of the top of your head you must know that the center of the outspread limbs will be in the navel and the space between the legs will be an equilateral triangle." [7]

How did he achieve this, or we can ask, how did he measure this 1/14 decrease? We see in his extensive notes in those piles of notebooks on the human body, he tries to better understand the joint of the shoulder, because he noticed that it doesn't move like the other joints. It kind of floats around in the shoulder, it doesn't just move up or down, like the knee joint. This joint can move up, down, forward, and backward. It can even rotate, but it still can lock in certain places. This is where he had used cadavers and assistants to measure, and then he noted each measurement in those notebooks. This is one key feature that a lot of people don't recognize or they choose to ignore this problem altogether. Most people have a problem here, because when they measure the arm length, where do they measure to? How do I know that this is what da Vinci would have or could have done?

There are several ways explaining the way to draw the Vitruvian Man; one of the most notable would be to turn the square 45 degrees on its end. Take a look at Figures 7A and 8A, and you can see that this would be one of the easiest ways to draw it, but is this the way that da Vinci chooses to use?

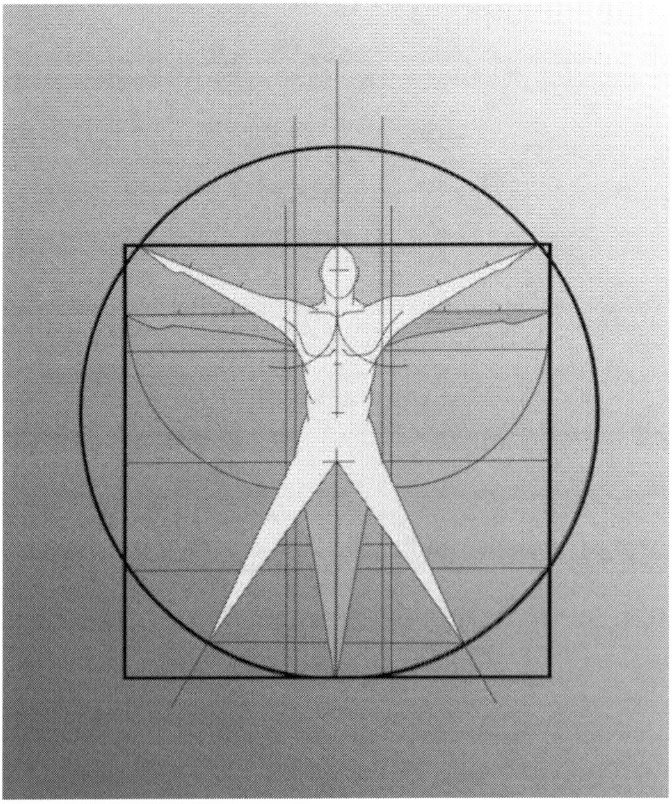

Figure 7A

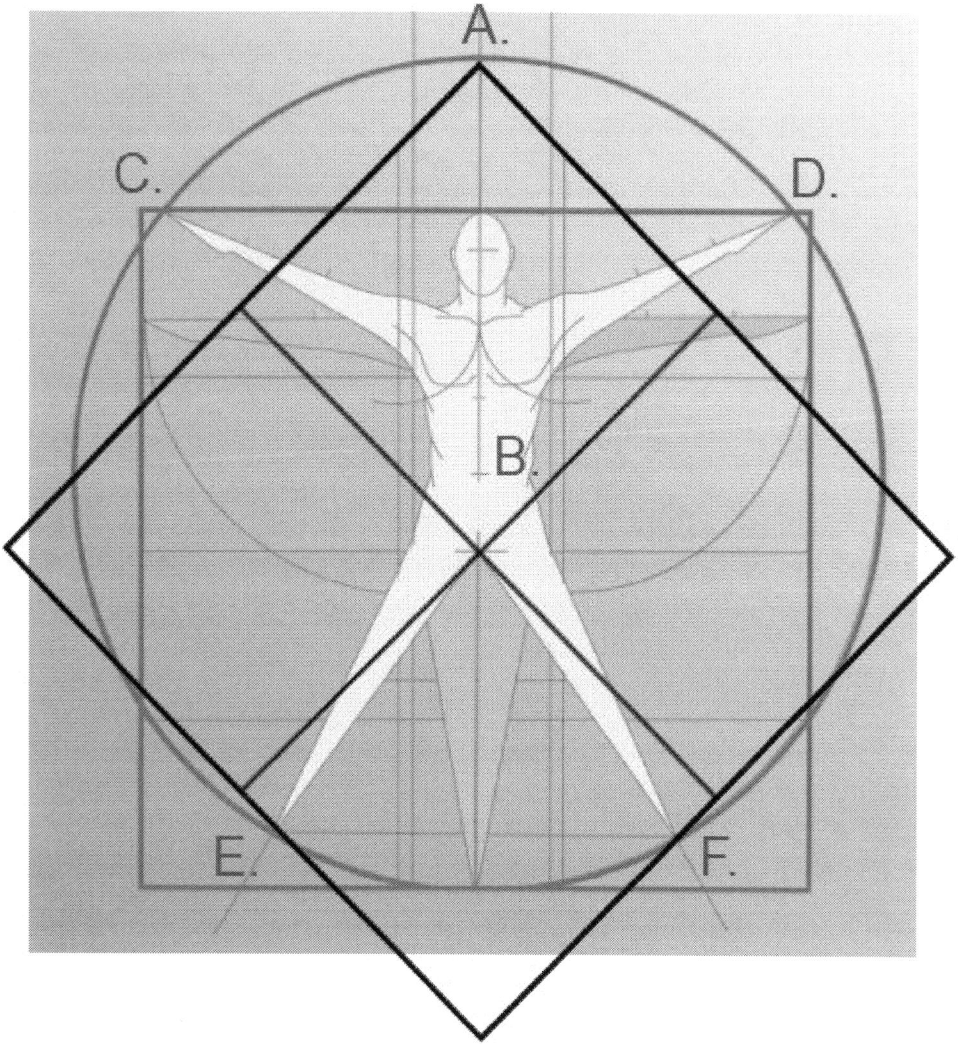

Figure 8A

Figure 7A is a version of the Vitruvian Man; and if we turn the square 45 degrees, it would look like Figure 8A. When it's turned, point A. would be the topmost boundary of the circle, and from there we can measure to the bottom of the square to find the diameter of the whole circle. If we divide that number in half, the center of the circle at point B. can be found. At points C. and D. we find the location for the hands; and at points E. and F. the positions for the feet are found.

This would seem to be the best way to draw the picture; but that's not how da Vinci works. There are flaws in this method; the biggest flaw would be that the square and the circle have different areas, and he was one that was obsessed with finding a way to square the circle; another would be that he didn't explain this method in the notes surrounding the drawing, and even if he would have started here with this method, I believe he still would have wanted to know, "Why does it work like this?" and "Does it apply to everyone?"

I think that's why he left off the square that would be turned; because he used other methods to solve this riddle. He may have solved the drawing first using this solution; but it's what he would have done after, that would be genius. I don't think that da Vinci would have just taken the word of Vitruvius, about a set of proportions for the human body; I think he would have wanted to prove that idea for himself.

I think he left us hints inside the drawing itself. If you notice that on his drawing he has two lines still drawn across the shoulders, as seen in Figure 9A.

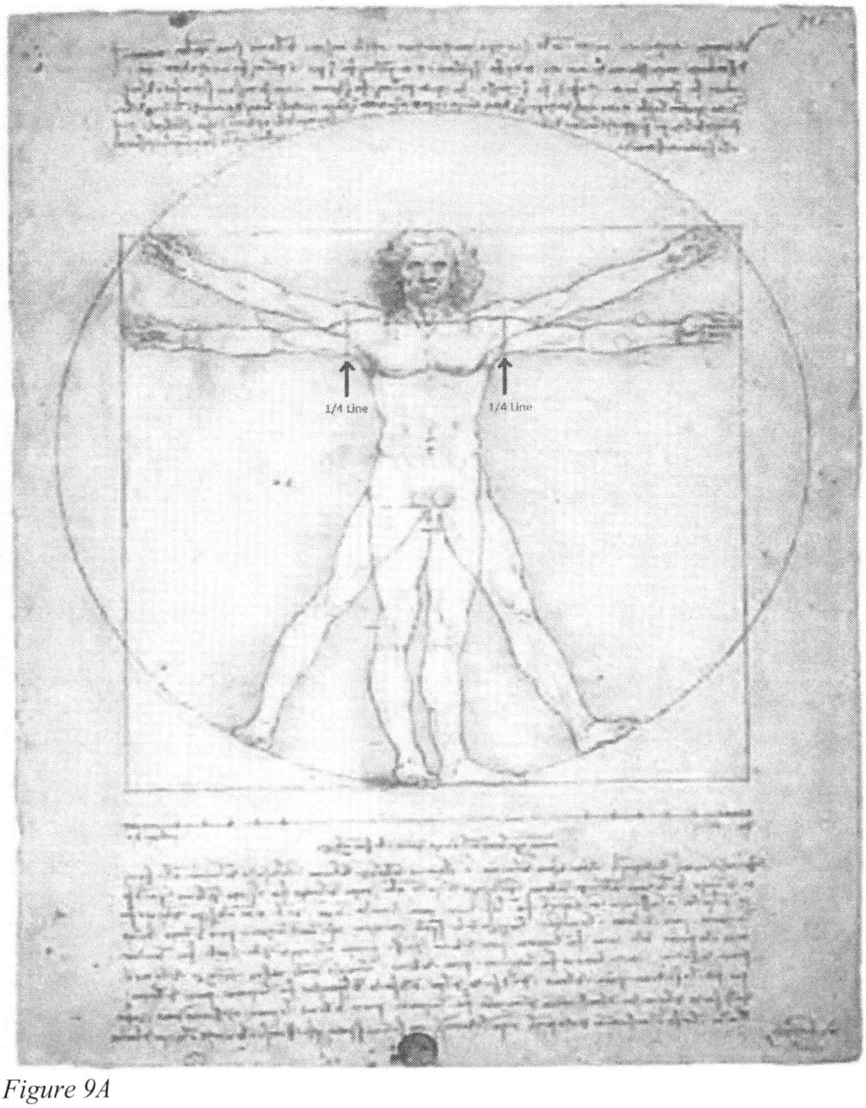

Figure 9A

These two lines are the ¼ Lines. If we draw these lines, the center line, the 1/6 horizontal line, and the ¼ horizontal line, we can see how he decreased the height better. If you take a compass and use the point of origin at the 1/6 Line and the ¼ Line at the shoulder, then draw an arc starting from the center line at the 1/6 Line and move the compass under the armpit at 7/25 from the top of the square. This is 0.28 multiplied by 5 inches, which is 1.4 inches from the top of the square. This is the inside arm rotation, as seen in Figure 10A.

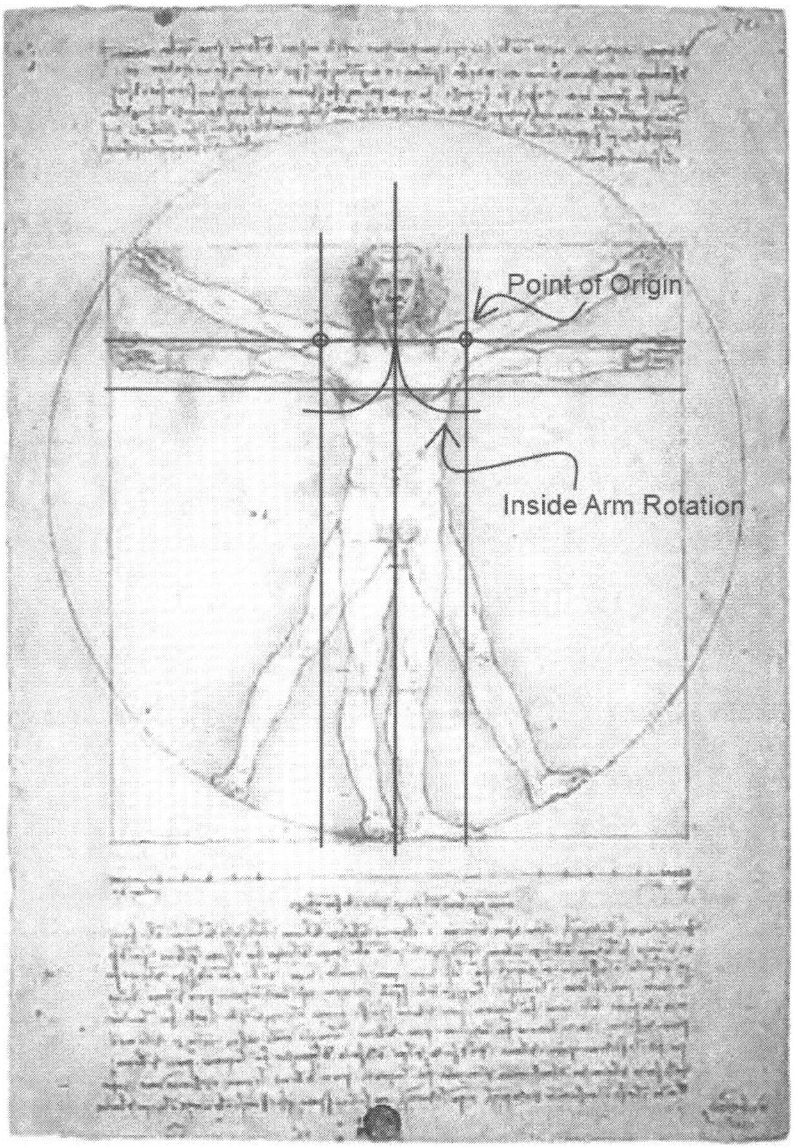

Figure 10A

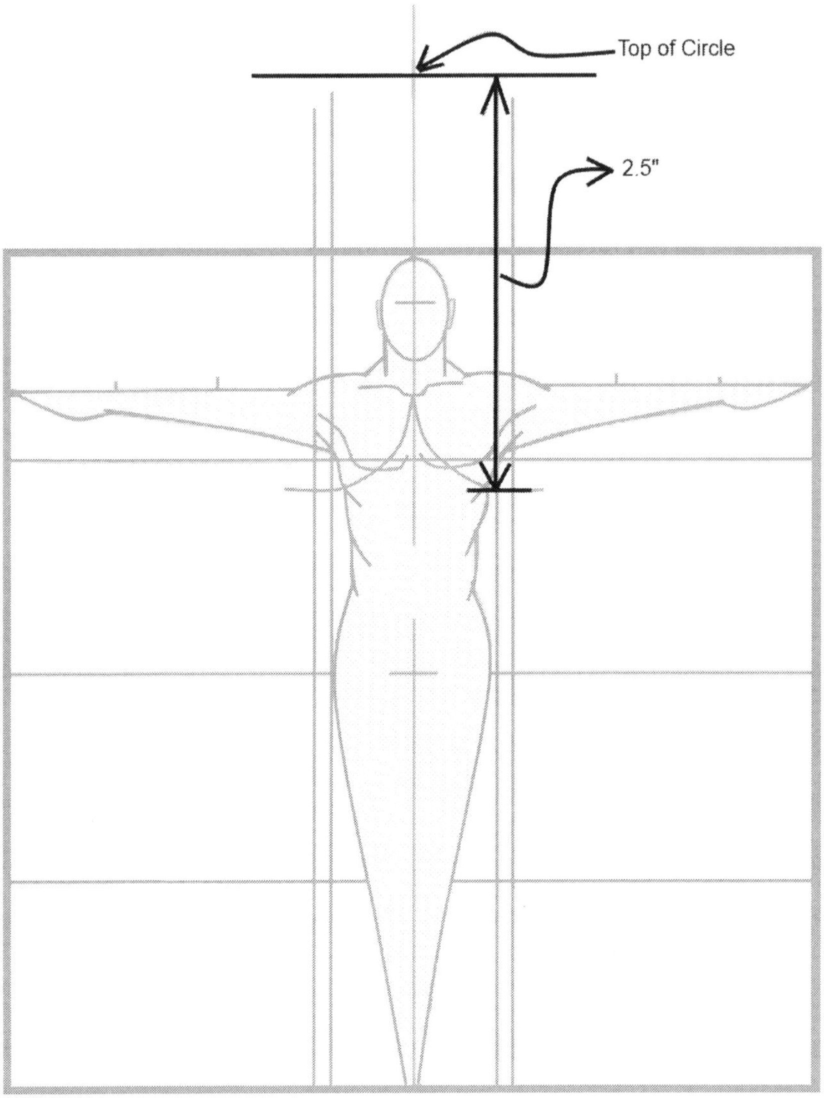

Figure 11A

Do you see how it's done so far? Place the point of the compass at the point of origin, as seen in Figure 10A, and then place your pencil end of the compass at the center line, just under the chin, and then draw the arc downwards until you reach under the arm.

Draw these rotations on your 5 inch square drawing now, measure the length of the arm from the center line out to the edge of the square. This will be 2.5 inches. You need to measure from the 1.4 line up the 1/5 vertical line, the arm length, which is 2.5 inches. This is the top of the circle. See Figure 10A.

Measure from the top of the circle to the bottom of the square and you find the diameter of the whole circle. The diameter for the circle for this drawing should be 6.125 inches and that would mean the radius would be 3.0625 inches. The center of the circle is the position of the navel. If we find the diameter of the circle this way, we don't have to know where the navel is placed first. Why is this so important? Well, let's say you want to draw a body without an actual body to reference where the arms will reach the top of the square. How do you know that the hands should touch the top at that certain point of the square? First you need to know how the arms will rotate, so you can measure the true length of that arm. Without knowing this, you're only guessing. What about if you want to draw a body without a navel? I know that sounds crazy, right? But if there was ever a reason to do that, at least now you'll know how!

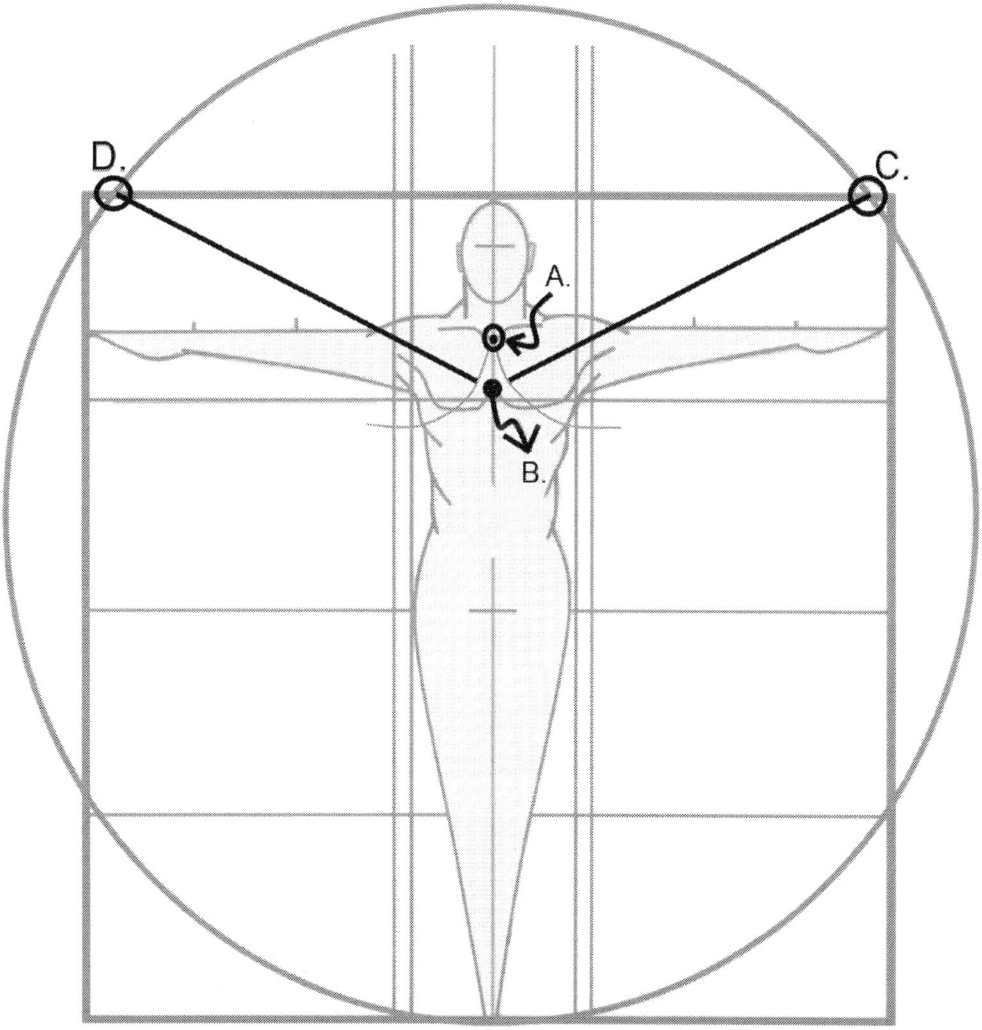

Figure 12A

Remember how da Vinci said "...decrease your height 1/14 and spread your arms till your middle fingers touch the level of the top of your head." [7] In order for us to accurately find where the hands touch, we also need to decrease the center line of the arms. Look at Figure 12A and you can see what I mean, at Point A. Measure down 1/14 of the magnitude of the whole body, or the height of the body, to Point B. For this 5 inch body it'll be 0.3571425 inch.

Draw a line from Point B. to Point C., and then draw another line from Point B. to Point D., now you know where the arms go and where the hands will touch the top of the square. If you measure these two lines, you will see they measure longer than the length of the arms from Point A. out to the side of the square where the hands originally touched. While the arm moves upward above the 1/6 Line, we have to only measure from the arm rotation itself. We have to take into account the floating joint of the shoulder and how it works.

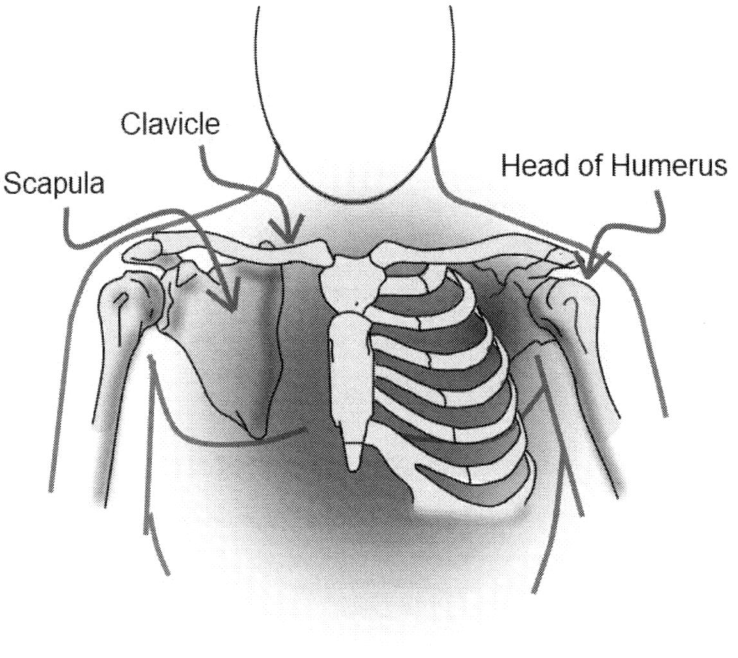

Figure 13A

In Figure 13A, we see three of the basic parts that make up the shoulder joint; the scapula, clavicle, and the head of the humerus. These three important parts are only functional with the addition of the many different ligaments and muscles that hold this joint together. The shoulder girdle, the muscles that surround the scapula, move the shoulder around unlike any other joint we have. It creates this multifaceted joint that can move our arms in almost any direction; and can even rotate the arm.

As the arm moves up; the whole system of this joint moves with it, therefore giving the arm a stretched look. Figure 14A shows how; not only does the arms move up, so do the scapula, clavicle, and all the muscles.

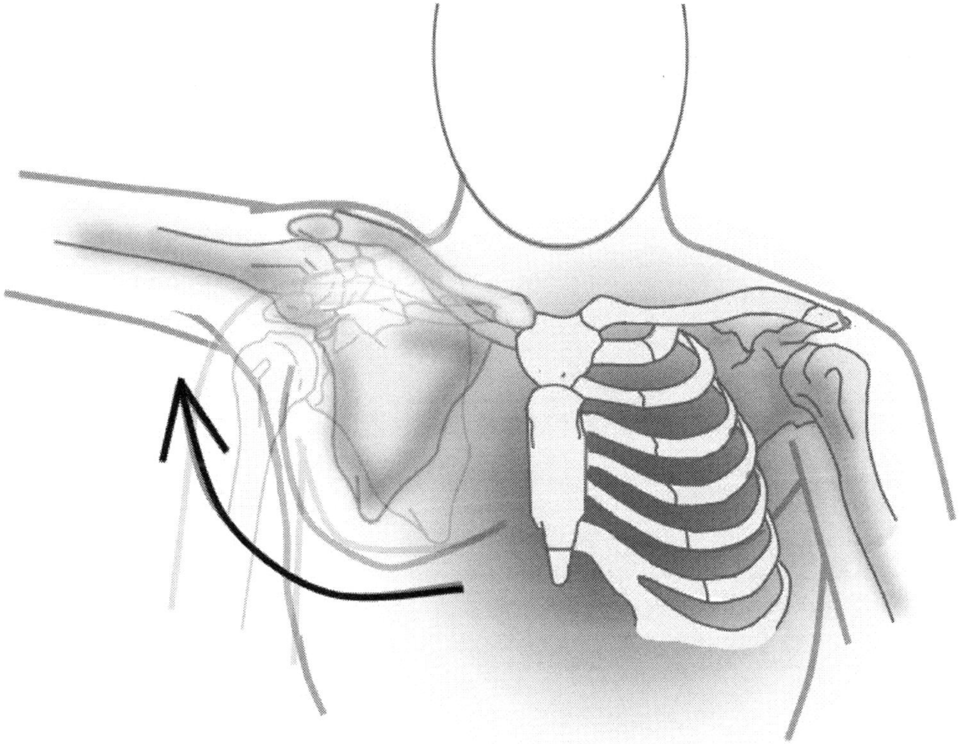

Figure 14A

We can see how intently da Vinci wanted to know how this mechanism worked; merely by looking at his drawings, like the one in Figure 15A and Figure 16A. As an artist in the 15th century; it would have been required that he studied the human anatomy from any of the latest treatises, and he would have studied it on his own. It would have been of the utmost importance that this subject becomes mastered; and da Vinci had a special talent when it came to anatomy.

You can see this rich detail in all his drawings; but most likely this one drawing in Figure 15A, was made after he drew the Vitruvian Man. The Vitruvian Man was drawn at his discovery stage in his art career; and he would have still been exploring all the different possibilities. He was still trying to find that one reason why this joint is different than all the other joints of the body; when he would have noticed how the arm seems to push away from the shoulder, but still remain attached just as well as the other joints.

When the arm does move up; it will push away from the shoulder joint, therefore making our arm measurement seem to grow in length. Look at Figure 17A and you'll see what to measure. You only measure from Point A. to Point B. and this will be the same measurement as the arm length when positioned horizontally.

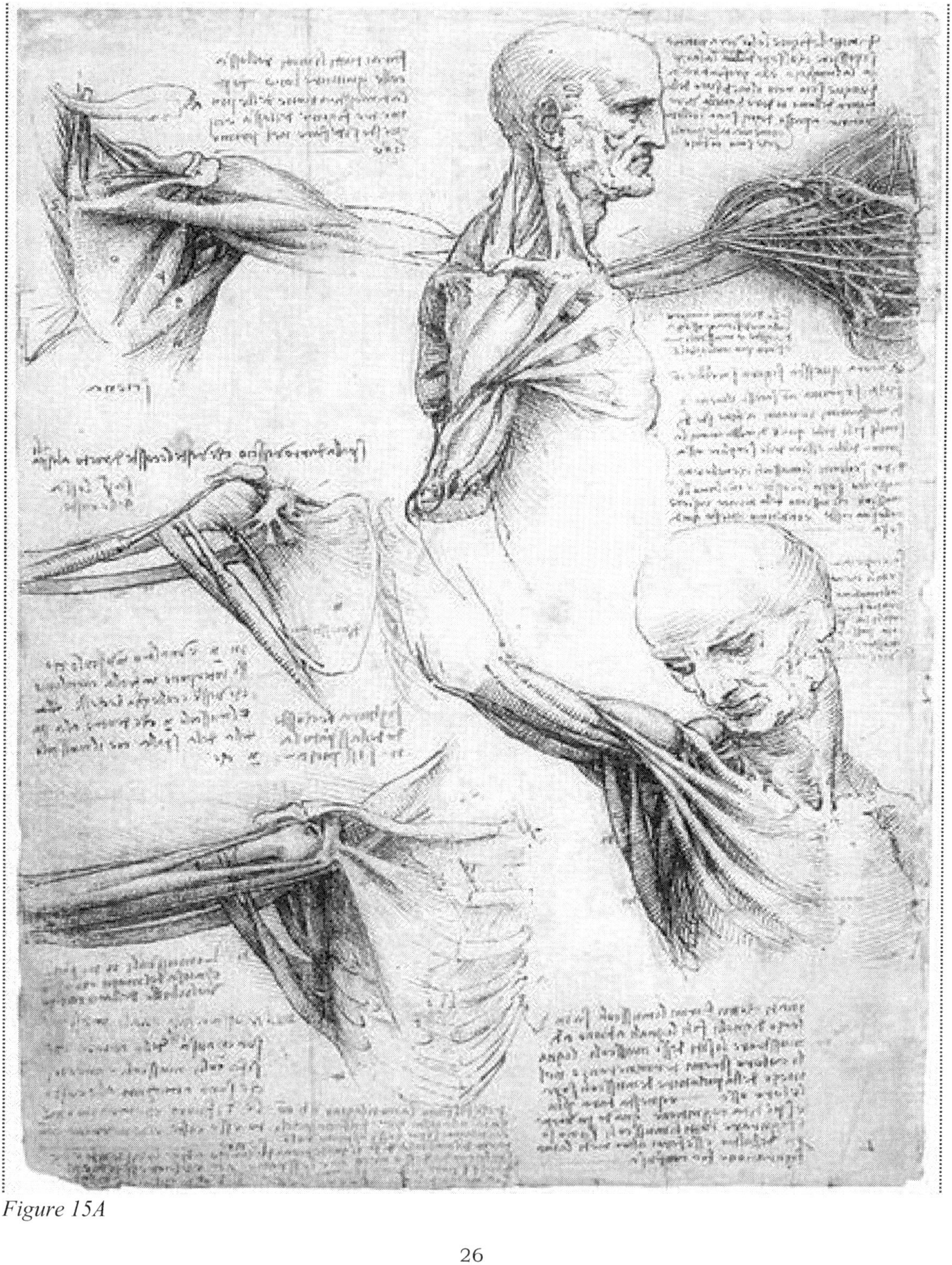

Figure 15A

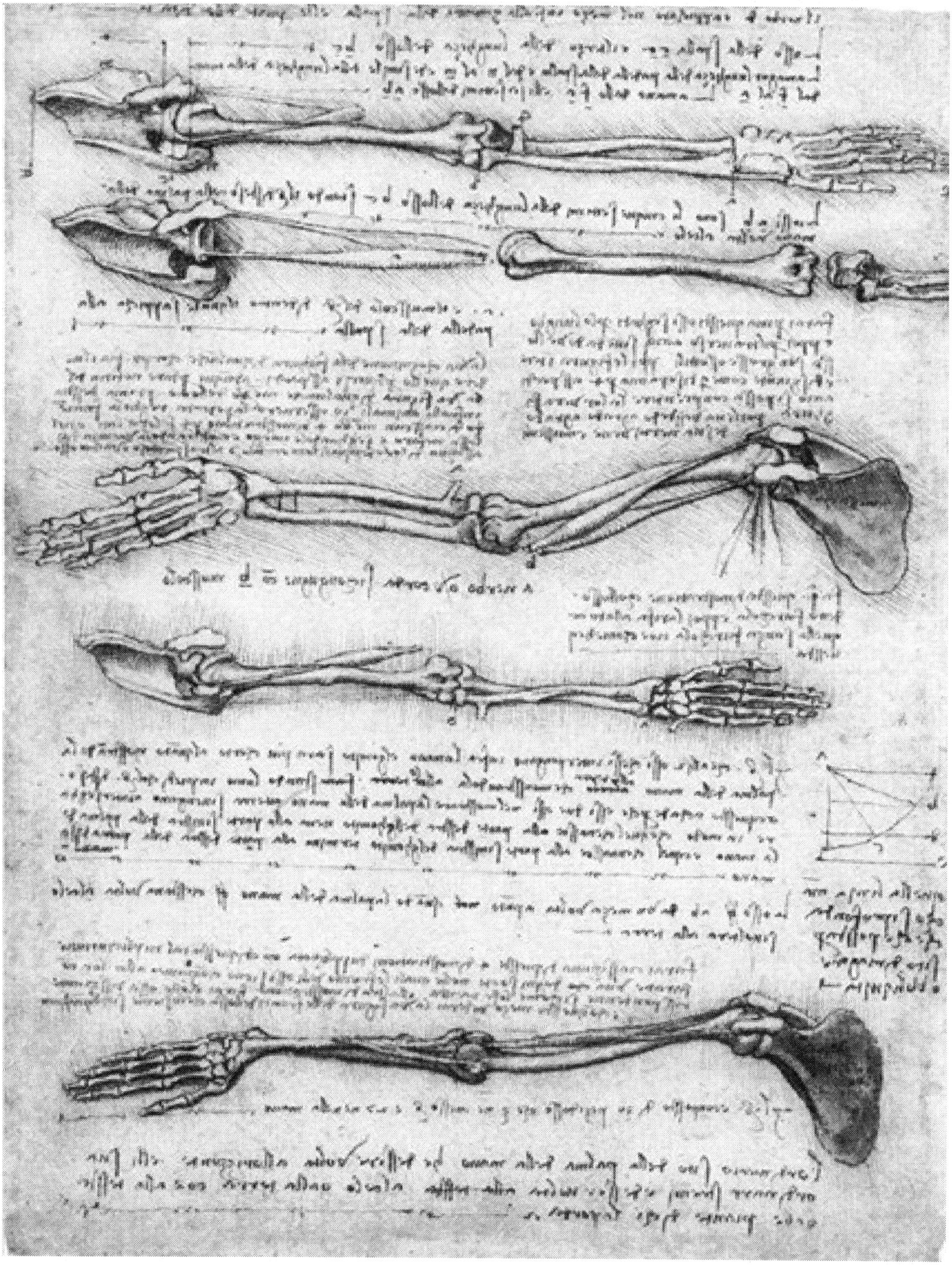

Figure 16A

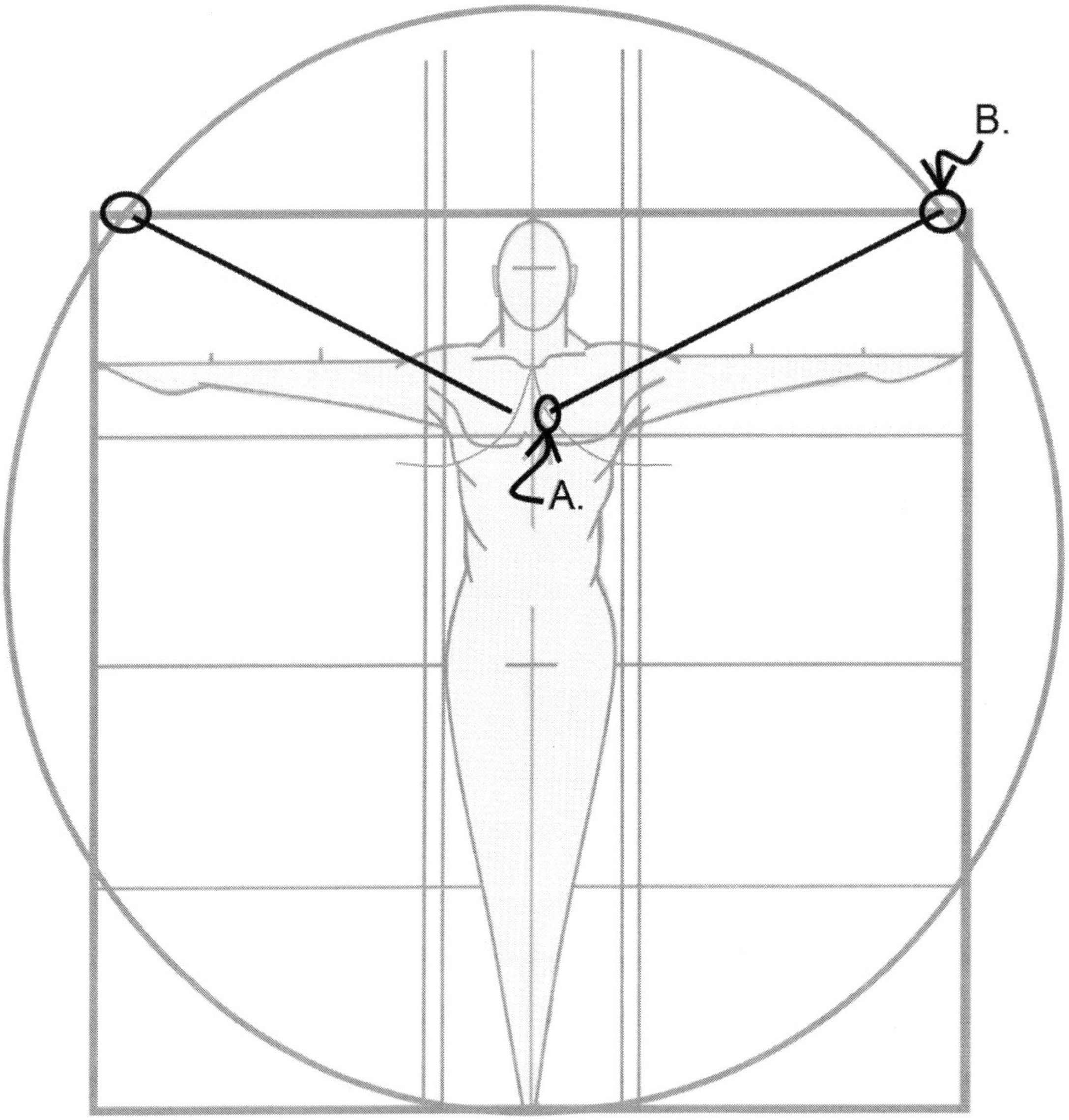

Figure 17A

Ok so we've moved the hands into their position, and now we can move to the other thing da Vinci said, "If you open your legs so much as to decrease your height 1/14..." [7]. How is that done?

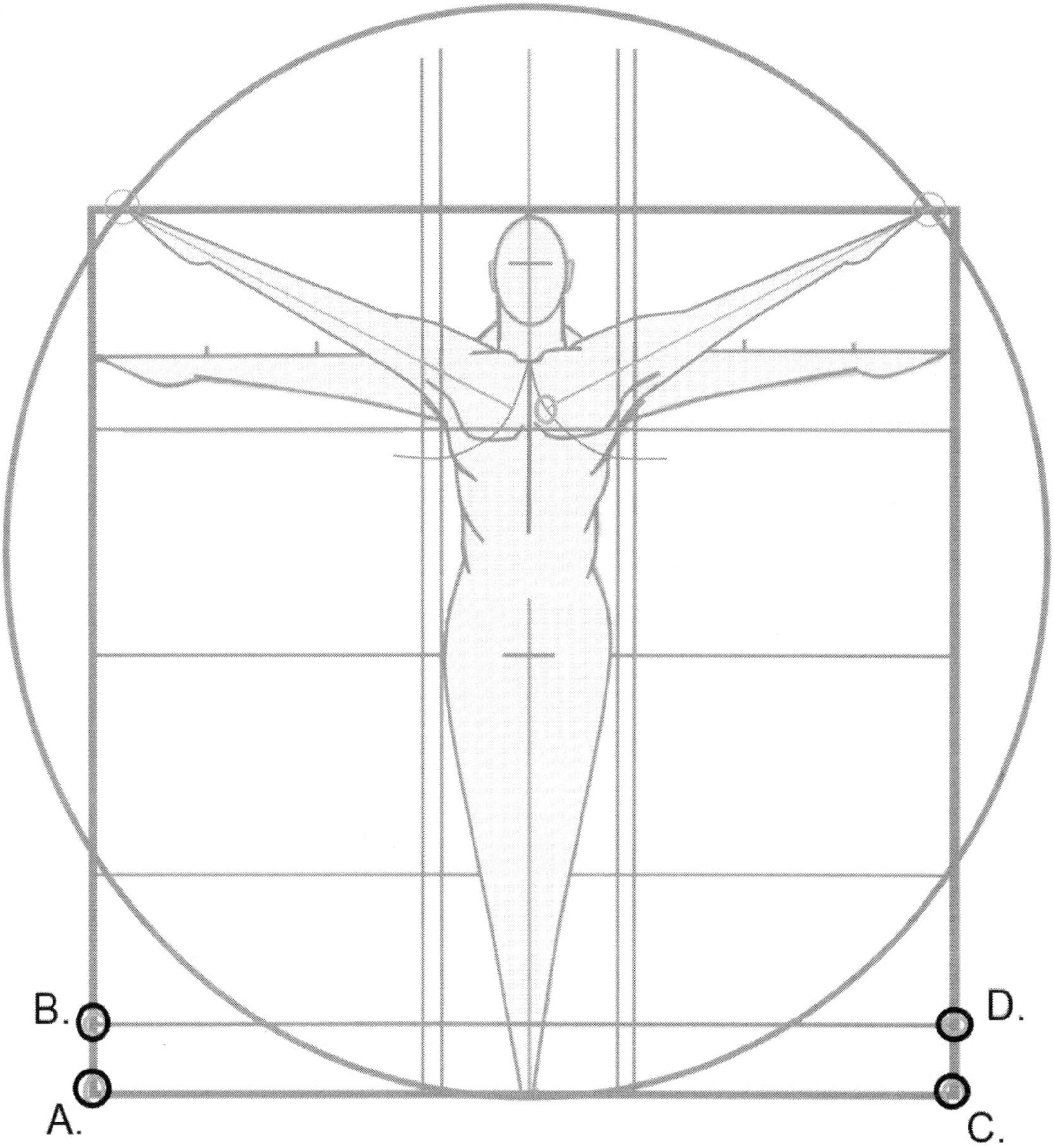

Figure 18A

You need to measure from the bottom of the square at Point A., Figure 17A, to Point B., the same measurement as before, 0.3571425, and then from Point C. to Point D., and draw a horizontal line from Point B. to Point D. Now move on to the next drawing, Figure 19A.

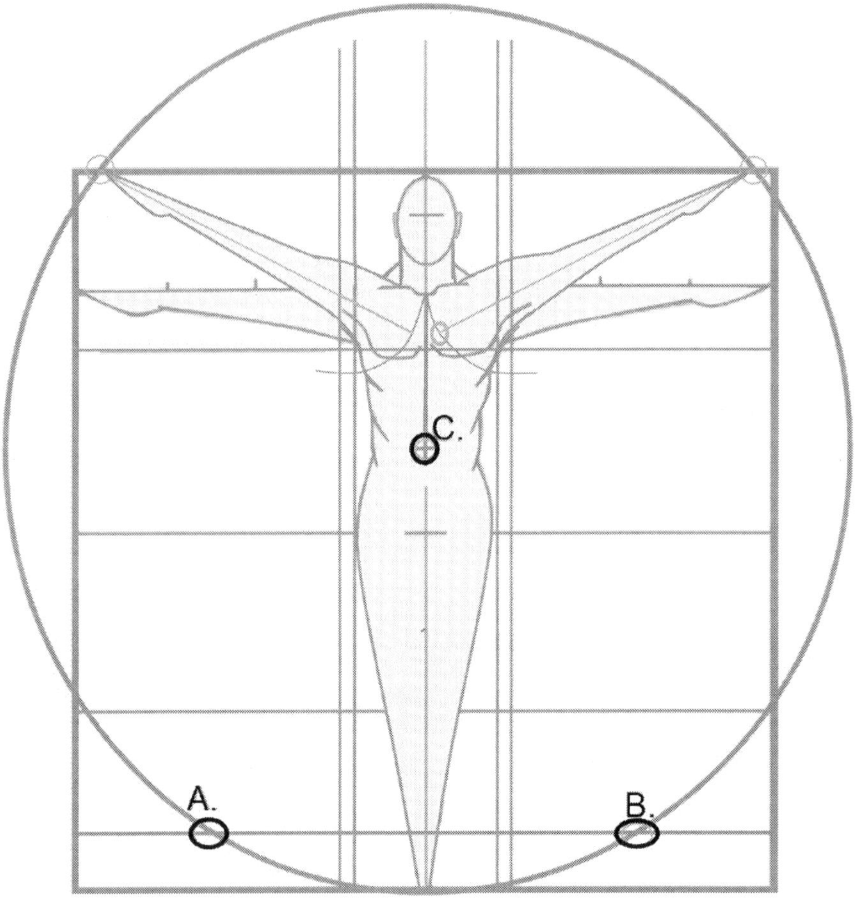

Figure 19A

Draw a line from Point A., Figure 19A, to Point C., and then from Point B. to Point C., to find the lines for the legs. See, that was easy enough, now we have all the necessary measurements and lines to draw that famous drawing; but there's one more way that he could have accomplished this same thing.

Vitruvius said, "Then again, in the human body the central point is naturally the navel. For if a man be placed flat on his back, with his hands and feet extended, and a pair of compasses centered at his navel, the fingers and toes of his two hands and feet will touch the circumference of a circle described therefrom." [4]. Let's stop here for just a minute, so we can understand this concept first. He states that the center of the body is at the navel. Could he have actually meant that what we call the center of gravity for a body is at the navel? He also said the hands and feet should be extended, but that doesn't mean that the hands have to be extended above the head, in fact, when you extend your hands above your head; the navel can't be the center of the body, then what could he have meant? I think this is where the genius of da Vinci understood that

Vitruvius meant the center of gravity for a human body is naturally the navel, not the center of magnitude.

What does the magnitude of the body mean? Magnitude is described as being the size of an object, so what object are we talking about? That's right; the human body is the object we are concerned with right now. The magnitude of the body would then be the height of the body. This same magnitude would also be the height of the square and so if we were to move the center of magnitude of the body, we would also be moving the center of the square that surrounds the body.

What about the center of gravity of the body? Is it still positioned naturally at the navel without any circle encompassing the body? Yes it is. The center of gravity is a force that acts upon the body in a static position. The center of gravity is where there's a sort of equilibrium between that body and the natural force of gravity. This would be separate than just the center of the body and it moves as the body moves. It's something that can't be seen, but it can be measured. It's like a balancing act between you and gravity, and if this center moves too far one way or the other, you lose your balance. I believe that's all Vitruvius was trying to say; that the center of gravity is naturally at the navel in the human body in an upright position, and I think da Vinci recognized this when he studied the books that Vitruvius wrote.

If you look at Figure 20A, you will notice that the center of the circle is also the center of the square, and the square is the same height as the circle. This does not mean that they have the same area, just the same size, width, or height, however you may want say it. This would be the center of the magnitude of both the square and the circle, and this is what it would be like without a body within either one. This is a key feature that needs to be recognized with or without a body, and it helps to see this without the body.

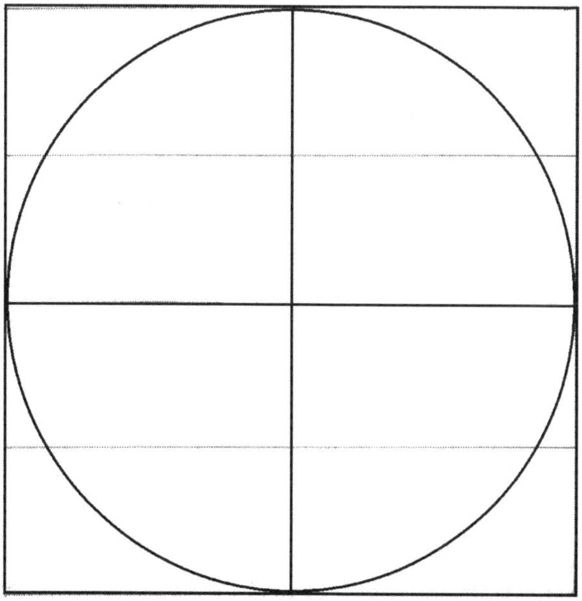

Figure 20A

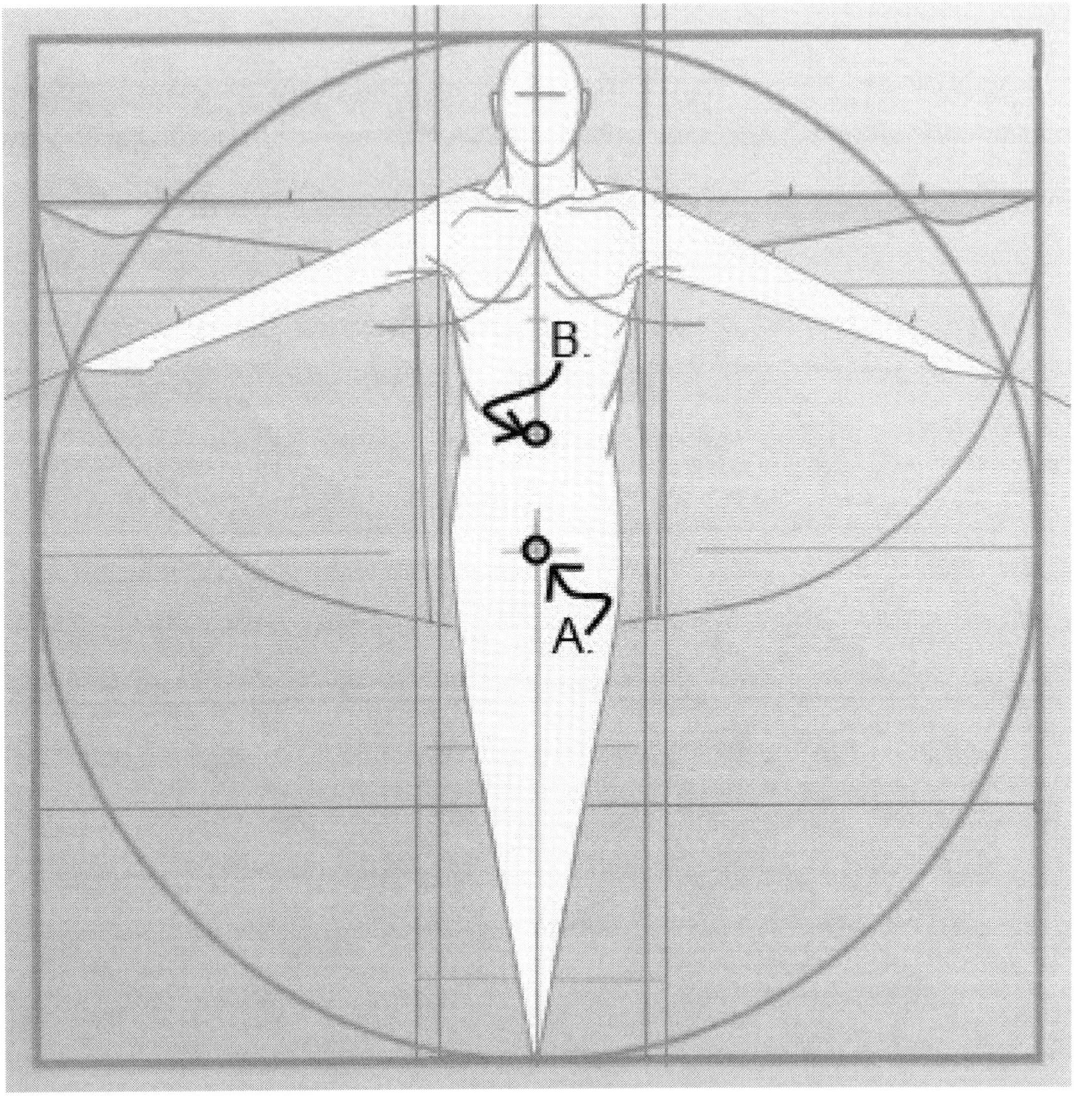

Figure 21A

Now look at the same thing, but with a body inside the square and the circle, as seen in Figure 21A. At point A, the center of both the square and the circle is at the pubic region. Point B is the center of gravity for the body and the navel placement. Those two points in a body in an upright position will almost always be different. Leonardo is the one who said that you can shift the center of magnitude; which is at point A, without shifting the center of gravity, which is at point B and we'll see in Figure 22A, point B remains in the same place, but point A moves up to point B, therefore shifting the center of magnitude without shifting the center of gravity.

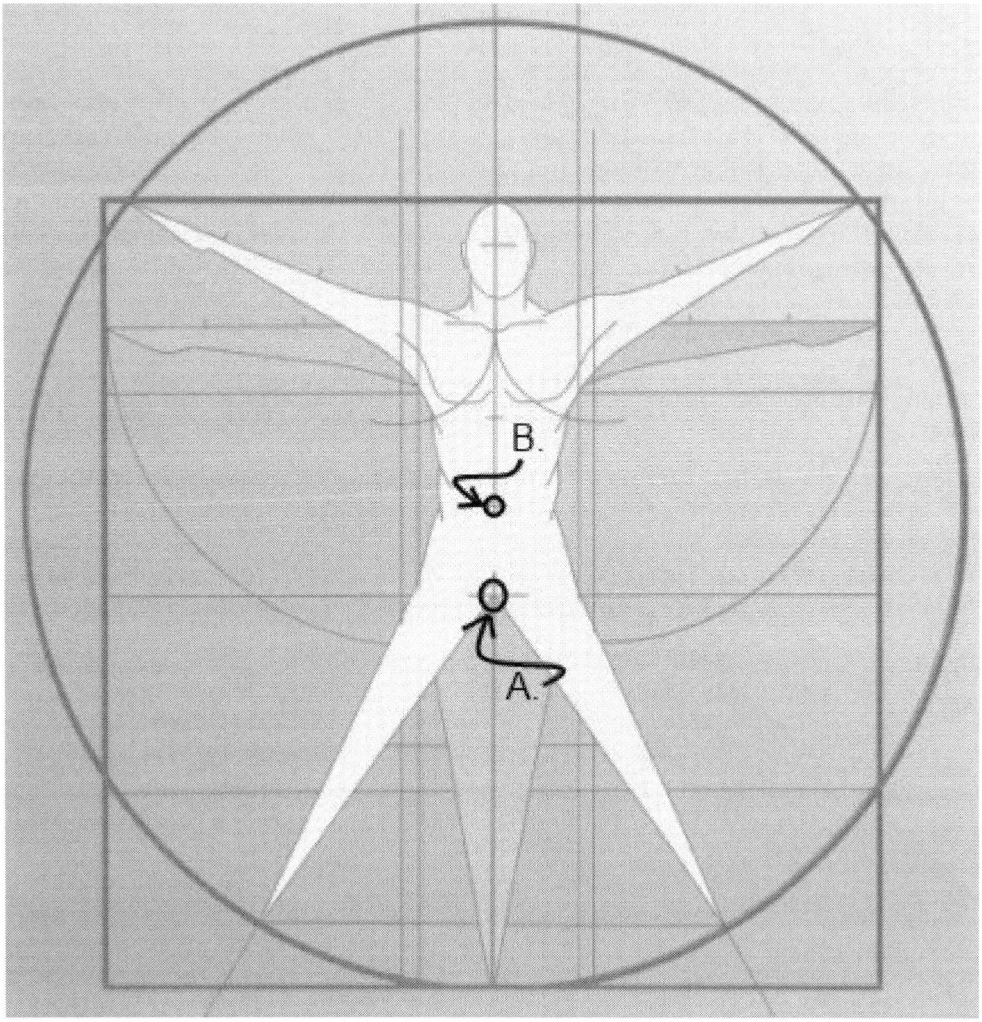

Figure 22A

Do you see how the center of magnitude for the circle moved from point A to point B and the center of the square didn't change and neither did the center of gravity for the body.

We know now what Leonardo meant by shifting the center of magnitude without shifting the center of gravity, but does it still meet the criteria Vitruvius described without breaking away from what he said? Here, let's look again at what Vitruvius described and compare it to the drawing, one item at a time. First, Vitruvius said the hands and feet need to be extended, and in the drawing, da Vinci accomplishes that. Second, Vitruvius said the hands and feet need to touch the circumference of the circle, not the square, and Leonardo did that too. Third, Vitruvius said, "For if we measure from the soles of the feet to the top of the head, and then apply that measure to the outstretched arms, the breadth will be found to be the same as the height, as in the case of plane surfaces which are perfectly square." [4] Did da Vinci achieve this? I believe he did! The position of the body under the position that touches the circumference of the circle is touching only the sides of the square, just as Vitruvius described. The final item that Vitruvius described, is the center of the body being placed naturally at the navel; and as described earlier, I believe he may have meant the center of gravity; and I also believe that da Vinci caught on to this idea, or he could have taken upon himself to expound on this idea when he trying to find a way to combine both ideas that Vitruvius described.

Combine both ideas in one drawing? Da Vinci did break away from what Vitruvius said; but only in a way that could combine both of those ideas. Is that the only thing different than what Vitruvius envisaged? There's another thing that da Vinci done with the drawing that makes it so unique. He wrote on the notes surrounding the drawing, "If you open your legs so much as to decrease your height 1/14 and spread and raise your arms till your middle fingers touch the level of the top of your head you must know that the center of the outspread limbs will be in the navel and the space between the legs will be an equilateral triangle." [7]

Ok, here's one of the problems I kept revisiting when I was trying to figure out how he done the drawing: why or how did he come up with the 1/14 decrease in height measurement? This is what I came up with: he didn't just come up with the measurement, he measured it first! I think he probably had an assistant lay down, and then he drew a square around that person with his hands stretched out to the side, and then he measured from the navel to the bottom of the feet, or the bottom of the square, to find the radius of the circle. He would then draw that circle and seen that, when the arms are moved up to touch the top of the square, it too would touch the circumference of the circle. Da Vinci could have also done it another way, too. He could have raised the assistant's arms up first, and then measured from the point where it touches the top of the square to the navel, and then used that measurement for the radius of the circle. Ingenious, isn't it? It's such a simple idea of how to find the radius; and it didn't require any sophisticated tools or knowledge to find it, but it took someone like da Vinci to actually see how to do it. Man he was smart!

Da Vinci would have also used the radius of the circle to find where he stretched the legs out to find an equilateral triangle. So now the only thing we need to do is to move the legs up. Since we know that he had someone to move their arms up, we don't need to worry about that. We measured up from the bottom of the square 1/14 of the whole measured height of the body or the square, and then we marked those points. Let's look at Figure 23A to better see what I mean. We measured from point A to point B; 1/14 of the height of the square, and then we measured from point C to point D to find an intersection on the circumference of the circle where the feet would touch.

Simply draw a line from point B to point D; this will give us a reference line to go by when we draw the legs. If you notice that we got to this same position when drew the earlier version; but with this one you will need the help of an assistant.

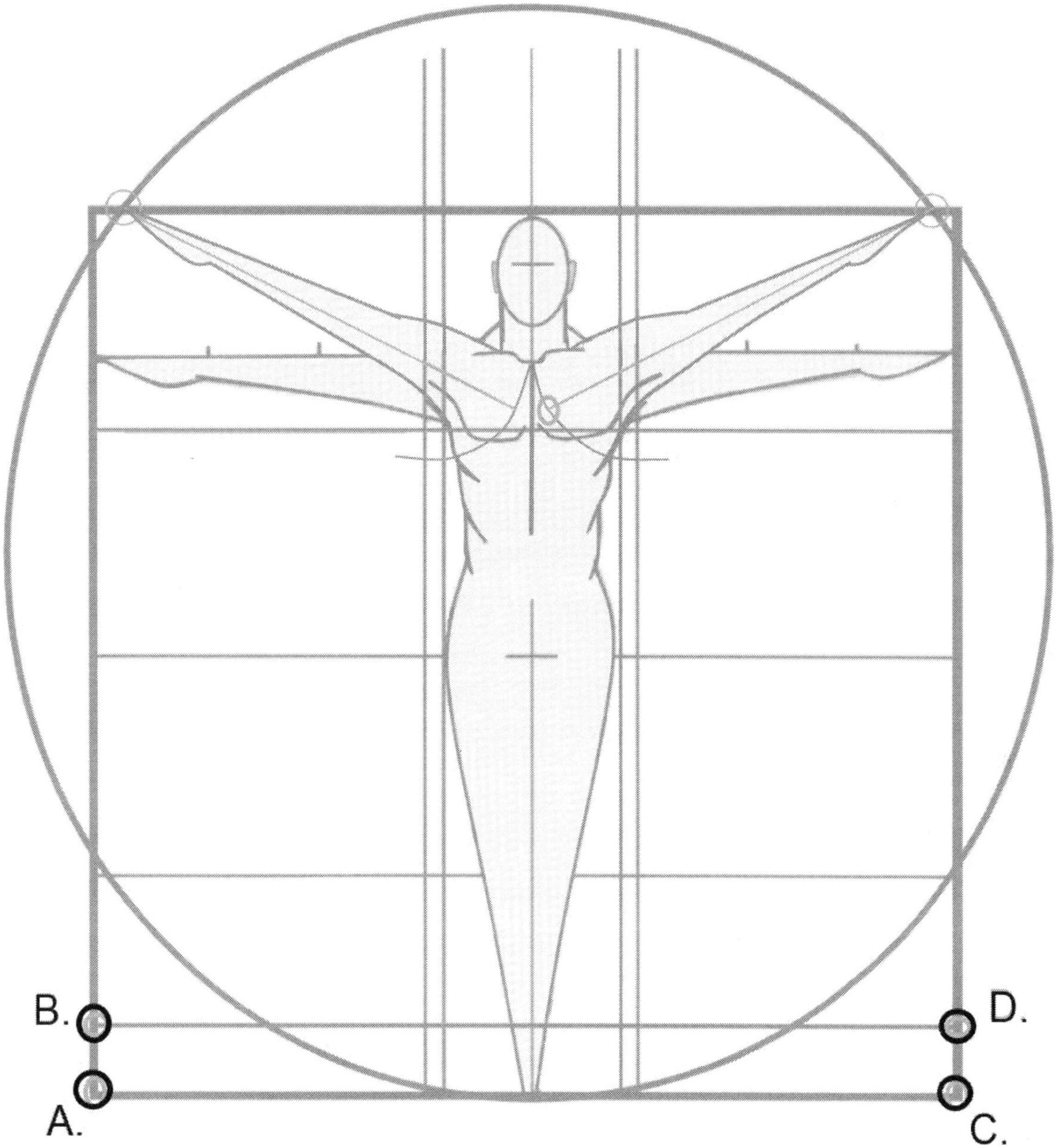

Figure 23A

The next thing we do is draw a line from those points on the circle up to the navel, as we can see in Figure 24A. We draw a line from point C; in Figure 24A, to point A and then from point C to point B; in Figure 24A. This is for the lines to draw the legs. I think instead of doing the measurement like this first, da Vinci could have used a straightedge with the radius marked on it, laid it parallel to the bottom of the square, and then moved it up to find where that measurement would intersect the circumference of the circle, and then placed the feet there.

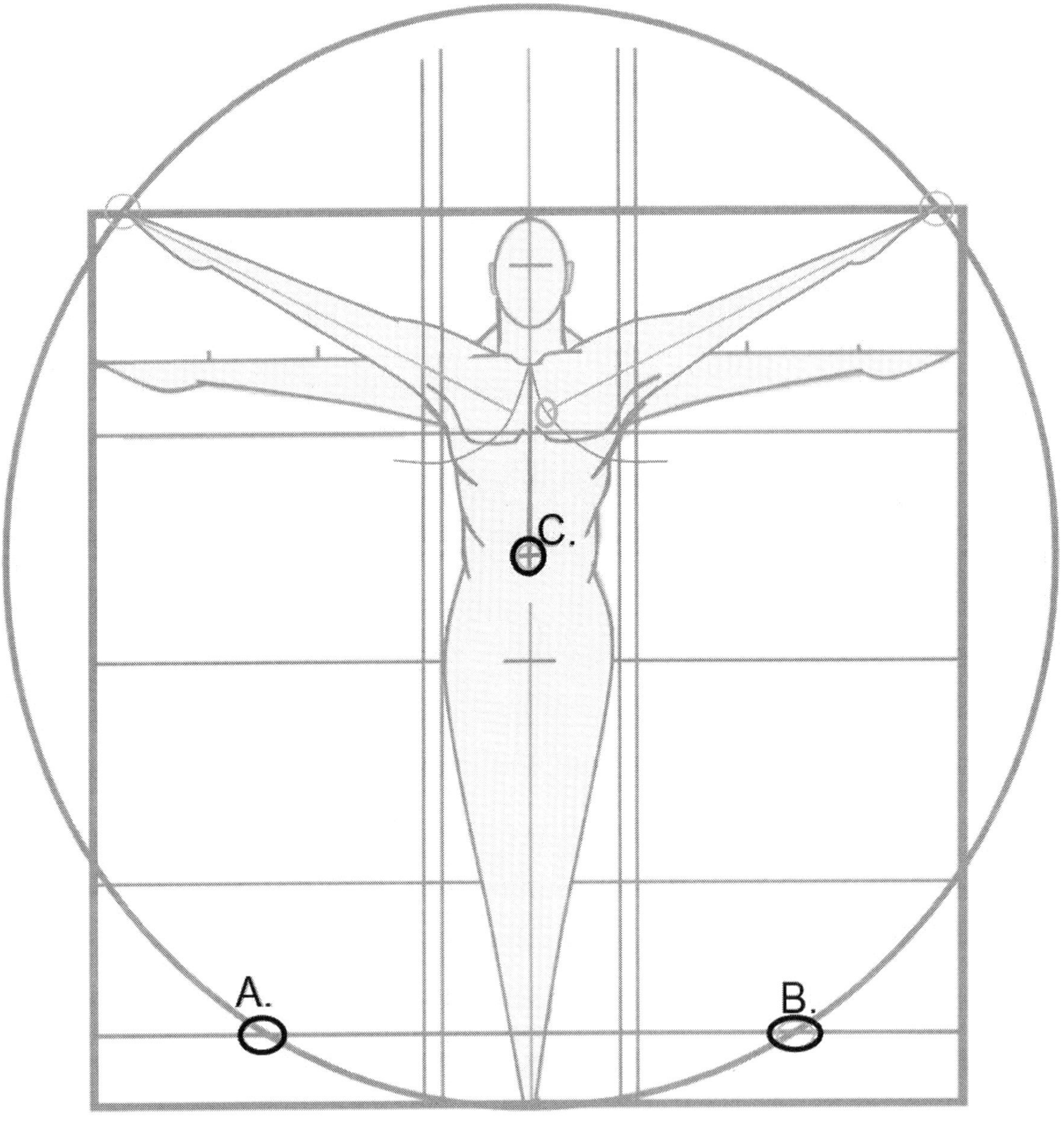

Figure 24A

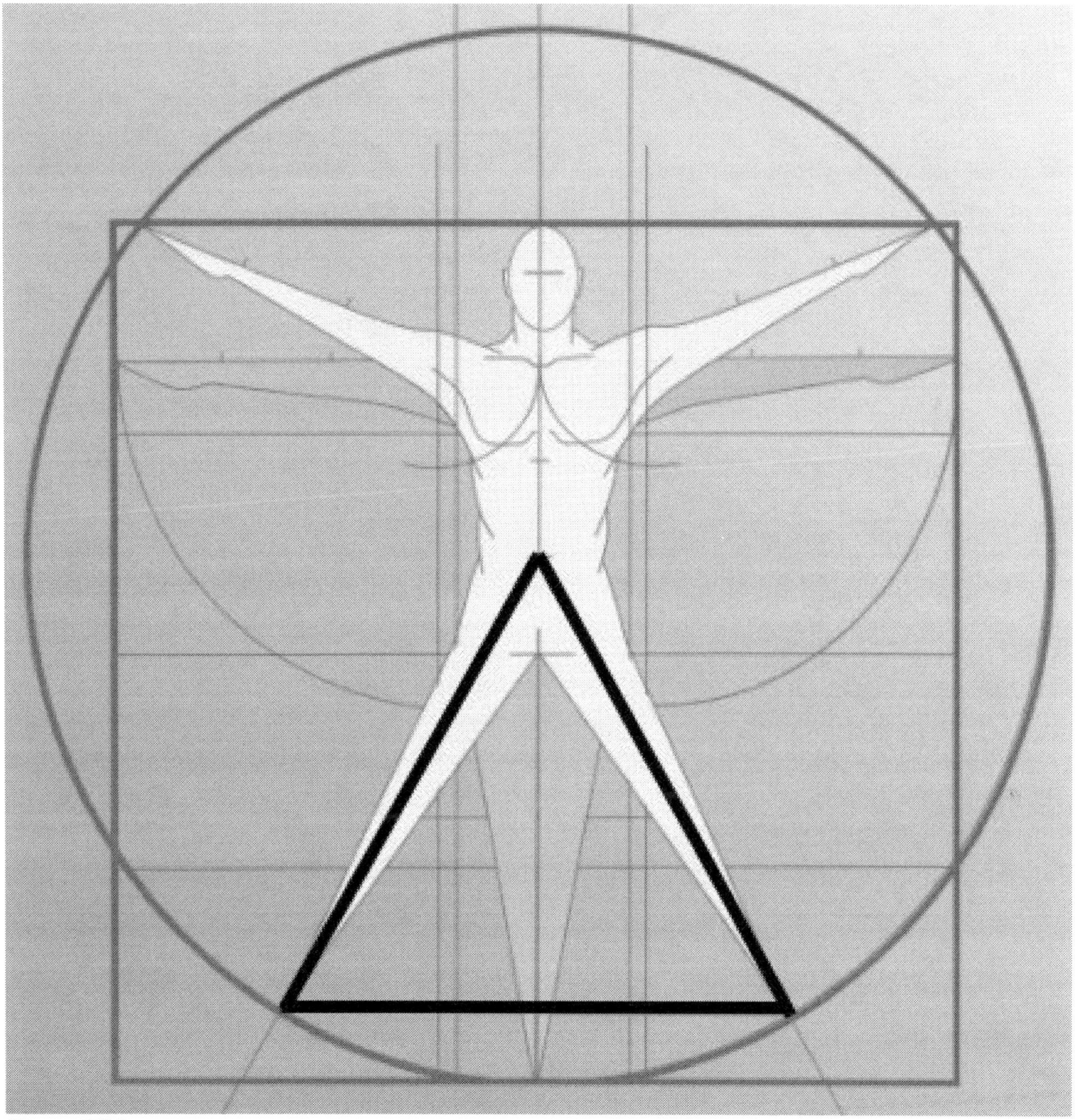

Figure 25A

Drawing the two legs would then make an equilateral triangle like the one seen in Figure 25A. Once he found these positions, he would have then measured from the bottom of the square to that line, and found that it would equal approximately 1/14 of the size of the height of the whole body within the square, finding the measurement by experimentation, not by calculation. He measured it first.

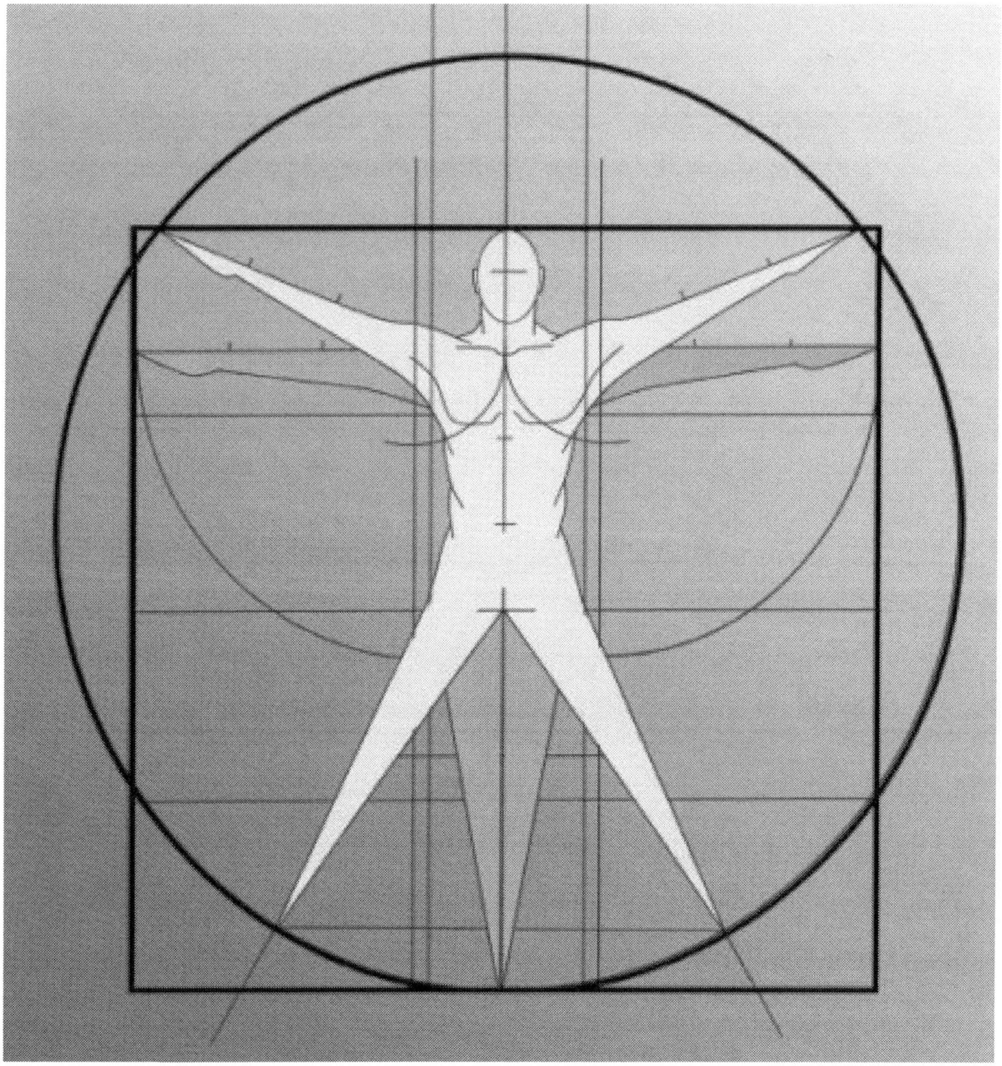

Figure 26A

This is how I believe da Vinci could have drawn his Vitruvian Man. It will work every time and it will work for any size. Now that we understand how he may have done it, we can explore the other ways da Vinci may have drawn the human body in a circle and a square.

I'm going to show you my own way of connecting the human body with the square and the circle in a way that neither Vitruvius nor da Vinci could have imagined. I've made several other versions of da Vinci's Vitruvian Man; to help us understand what he may have been thinking, showing that there was a process behind his masterpiece.

Here's a little taste of what's to come. Instead of trying to keep the body inside the square and the circle, we're going to push the envelope a little, maybe in the same way da Vinci did.

My Da Vinci Man

My Vitruvius Man is more inspired by da Vinci than Vitruvius, because da Vinci took what Vitruvius described and then added to it. He added his own research; this idea of a universal set of proportions would have grabbed any artist's attention at the time. The human body at this time was still such a mystery; most artists would have tried to combine a spiritual belief in their design, hoping to find a way to show how the human body would be a cosmic map to everything. It was da Vinci that would eventually take the spiritual design off the table, and he would describe the foundation on which every human body is designed by nature.

He explained it in a way that Vitruvius had not imagined, so now I will add to what da Vinci explained, and I will call it the Da Vinci Man. I believe that this series of five different, but interconnected proportional men; is necessary to explain how da Vinci could have seen a pattern in its form, a pattern that could only be from nature's design. I will begin by explaining a starting point first and then we'll build on it to form all five designs. In my measurements I will use a more related type of measurement with inches, instead of using cubits, palms, or fingers.

First, let's begin with the same drawing that's in Figure 5A.

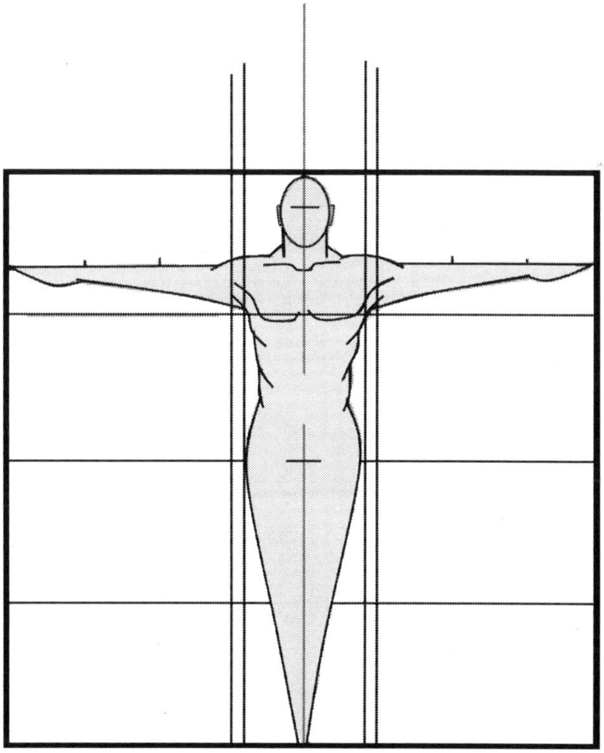

Figure 5A

Draw a circle with the center at the same center as the square.

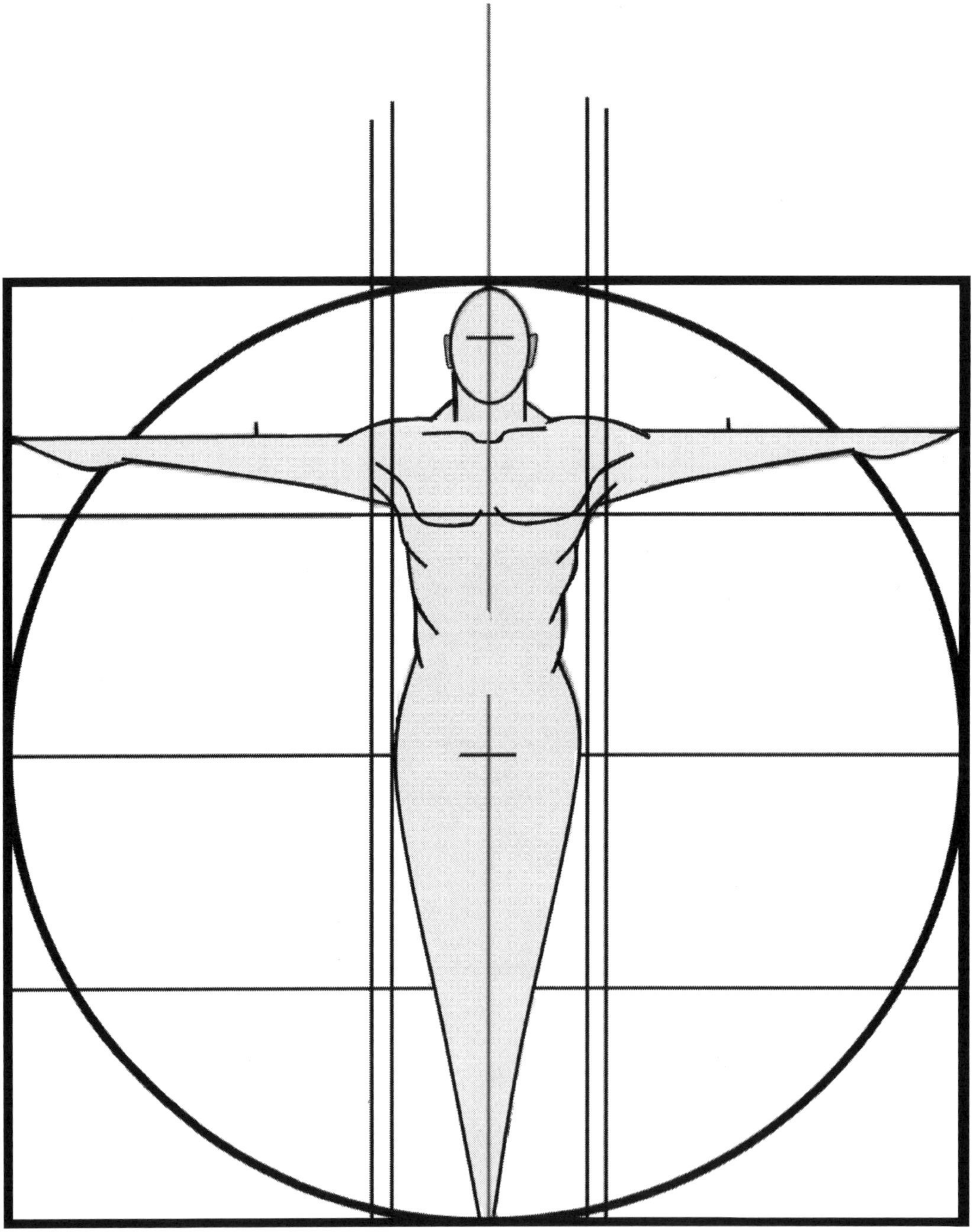

Figure 1B

As you can see, the circle is completely inside the square. It does enclose the head and feet. It does not, however, enclose the arms, so we need to make an adjustment in the arm position. Now we draw the arm rotation under the 1/6 Line only; to draw the arm positions, use a compass with the point of origin at the 1/5 vertical line on the 1/6 horizontal line. Start where the arms touch the square and then draw the line down to touch the legs. As seen in Figure 2B.

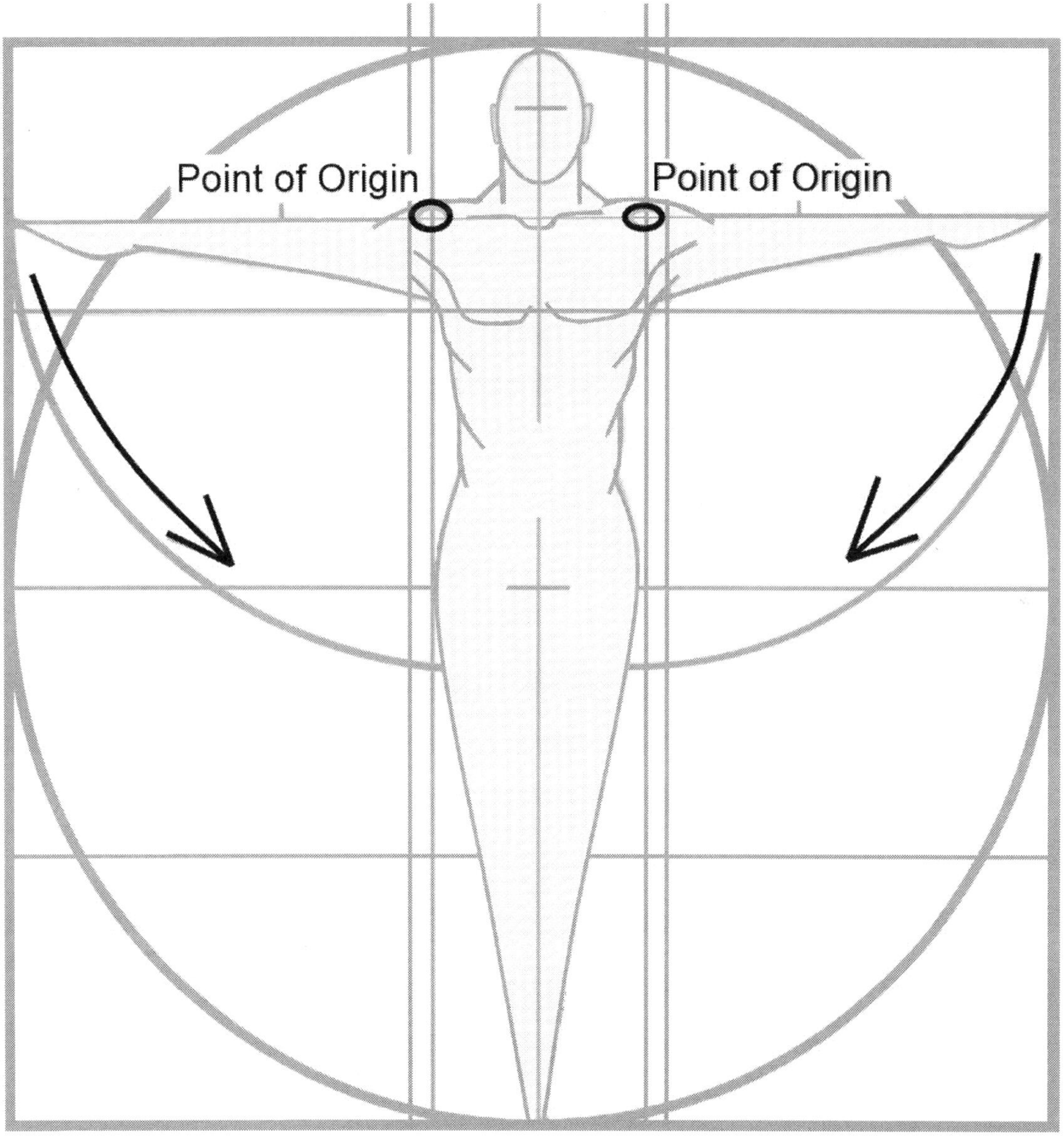

Figure 2B

Move the arms down the rotation until the rotation crosses the whole circle, this should be at around 1/3 of the square, from the top. For the 5 inch square, it will measure 1.666 inches, but instead of ended the line there, let's extend the line it touches the square. It will cross the square at 1.7416 inches from the top of the square. As seen in Figure 3B.

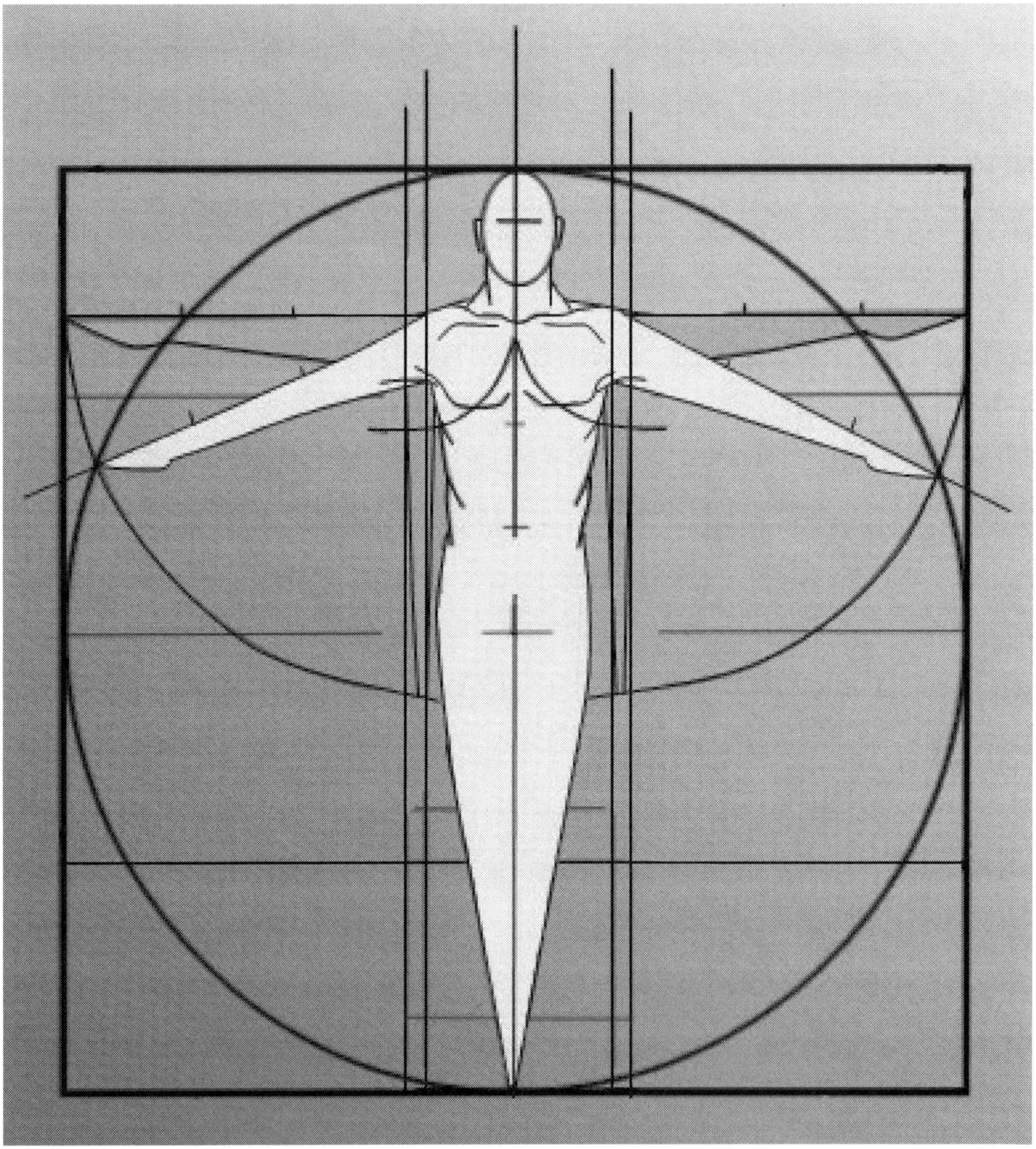

Figure 3B

This is my Da Vinci Man #1. This would be a perfect example of what a lot of people would first think of after reading what Vitruvius wrote. It may have also been a perfect starting point for da Vinci. It is a man within both; a square and a circle, but the navel doesn't seem to be in the middle of the body. These examples are steps in better understanding the secrets held by the Da Vinci Man, and once we better understand it, then we can see how the secrets can reveal the different proportions of each individual person. We will be able to see how each one relates to each other in the series; and then we can simplify this relationship into some simple equations, that will help us find those general features that make us look like we do.

If this was really the starting point for da Vinci; I could just image him setting at an easel or desk, toiling over what would be next. Without the navel in the center for both the square and the circle; then either his method or measurements were wrong, or he still had to find another way of fitting the body within both. He probably would have then tried to gather more measurements from live models, having them posed in different positions, measuring every single body part, and then comparing each part to see if there were any common ratios. This may give him a better way to see how a real body would move.

I think at some time while measuring his subjects; he would have seen that the best way to clearly see this movement would be to have the subject lie on the floor and draw a square and circle that would enclose his subject. It would have given him the perfect opportunity to see where to stretch those arms; this would also lead him to see that while trying to keep the circle and square connected, he would still have to push the circle outside the square.

His next reasoning may have been that if you wanted the center of both to be at the navel, then he may have to draw a circle with the same area as the square. This might move the center to the middle of the subject; therefore creating a more perfect union of the three, the body, the square, and the circle.

This would have seemed like an overwhelming task for most people, especially for those living at the time he drew the Vitruvian Man. Finding the same area for a square and a circle would prove to da Vinci that with the two most basic forms of nature, we could also find a common thread for the human body.

To find out how he found this common thread; let's move on now to the next Da Vinci Man, and put aside all of your preconceptions of how the human body works and let me show you the next step into my evolution of my Da Vinci Men.

For the next Da Vinci Man, begin with Figure 2B, except without the whole circle, as seen in Figure 4B.

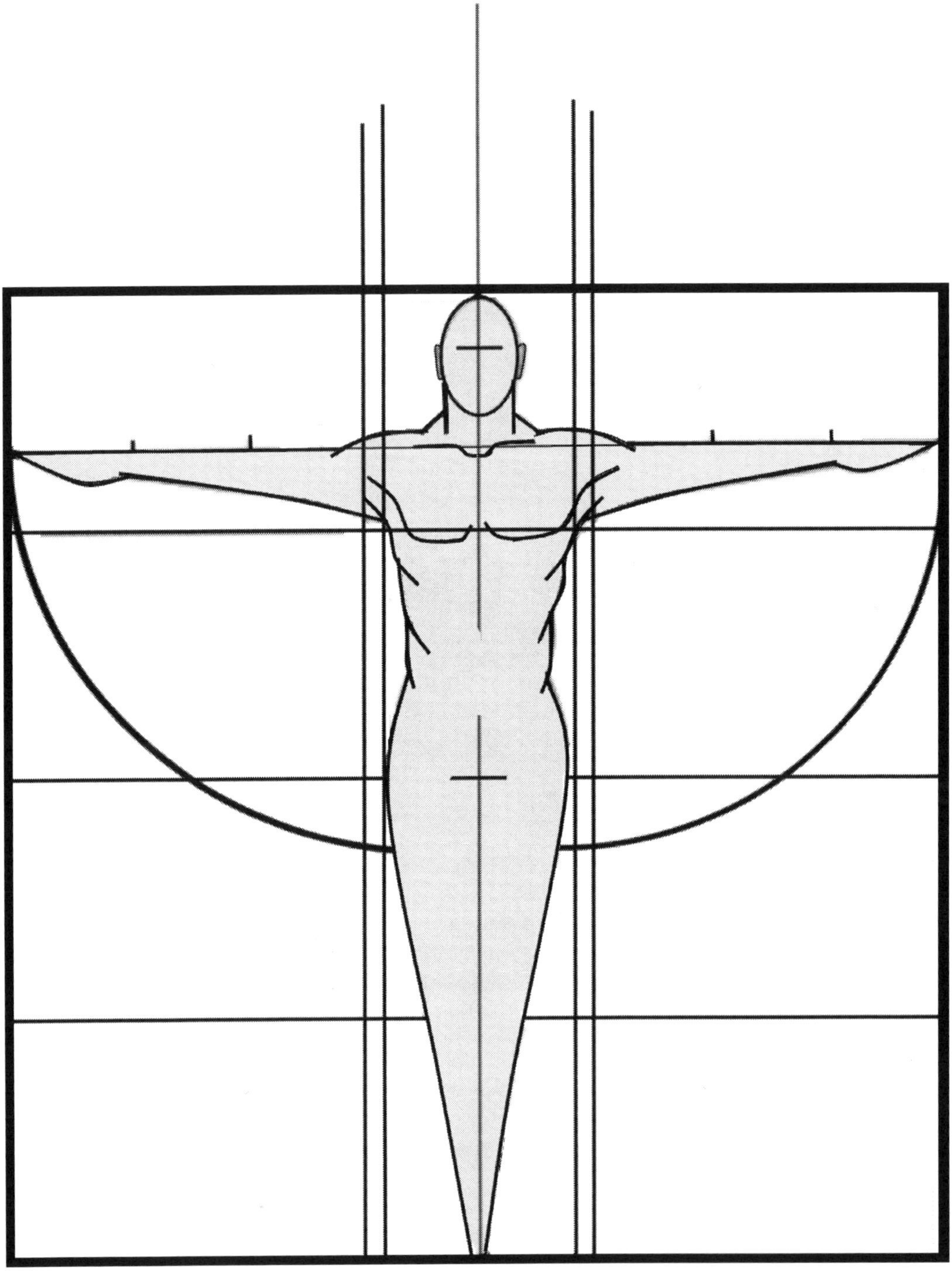

Figure 4B

Measure above the square approximately 1/8 the size of the height of the square or body height and mark that point. We could make our measurements from this approximation and it would lead to an approximate equilibrium of the circle with the square, but through trial and error experimentation, I have found a better approximation. You will see later why, but for now measure up from the square 0.642 inches. Even this approximation could be more precise, but for now we'll use this measurement. See Figure 5B.

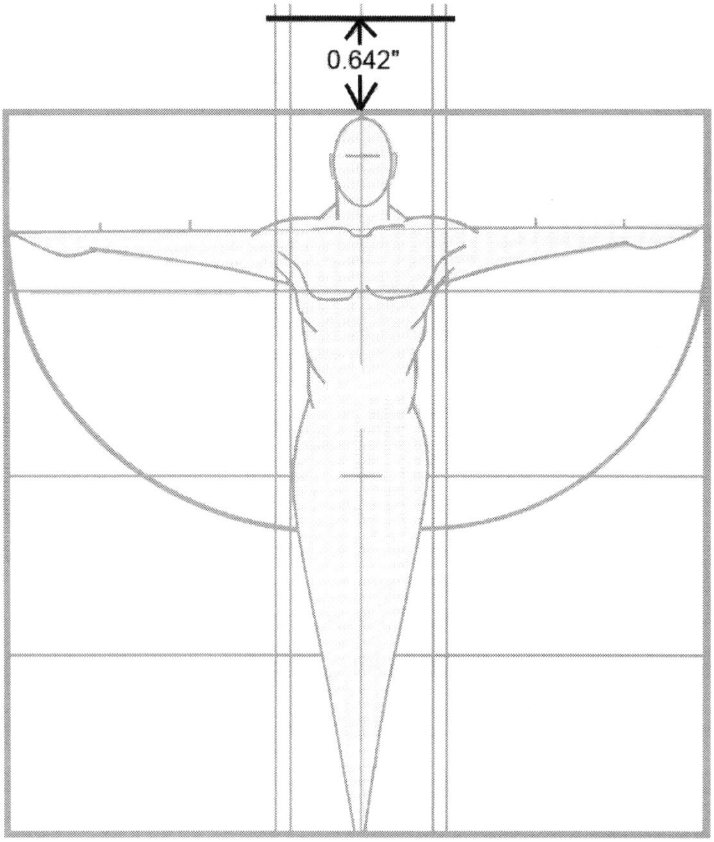

Figure 5B

You will need to measure from this point to the bottom of the square to find the diameter of the whole circle. For a 5 inch square, the diameter will be 5.642 inches and the radius will be 2.821 inches. Draw the whole circle. Now move the hand positions down the arm rotation where the whole circle passes through it. For the 5 inch square the arms should be at 0.9562 inches from the top of the square, as seen in Figure 6B. The navel will be positioned just above the center of the circle at 2.821 inches. This is where da Vinci may have noticed that the navel doesn't always remain the center of the circle; he would have noticed that the distance between the top of the circle and the square, seemed to have some kind of correlation with the way the center of the circle moves above the pubic region.

The distance between the top of the square and the top of the circle is 0.642 inches and the distance between the center of the square and the center of the circle is 0.321 inches. This would mean that as the whole circle increases in height "n" inches, the center moves half that distance. Example: 0.642 inches/2 = 0.321 inches. This correlation can be seen throughout all the different ways the body moves within the system of the circle and the square.

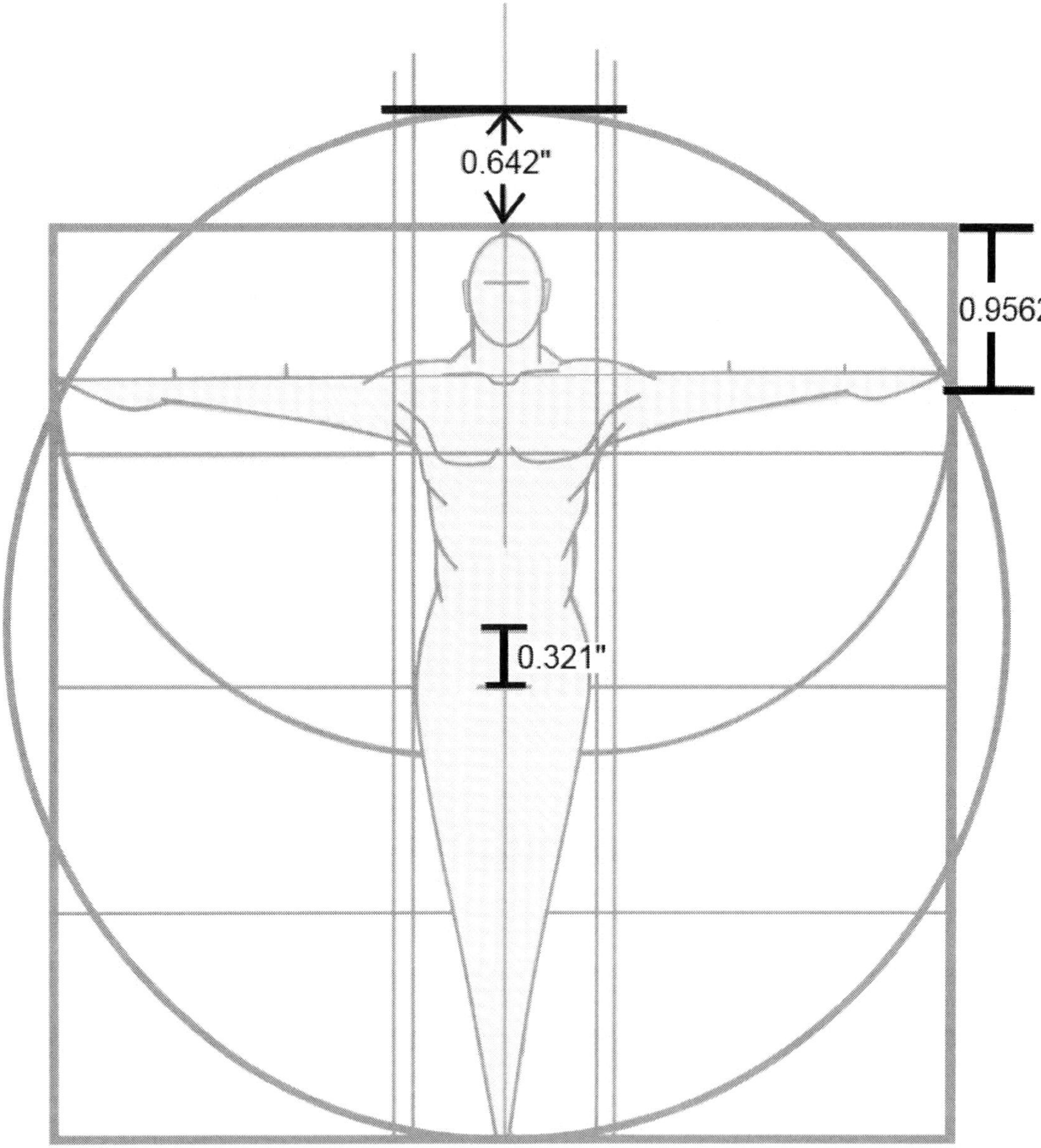

Figure 6B

This would have also been the moment da Vinci found an approximate equilibrium between the square and the circle. We'll concern ourselves with the other secrets and other relative similarities later after all the Da Vinci Men are completed. It is then when all the similarities can be explained. For now we can find an equilateral triangle, draw a line from the center at the top of the circle to the corners of the bottom ¼ Line of the square.

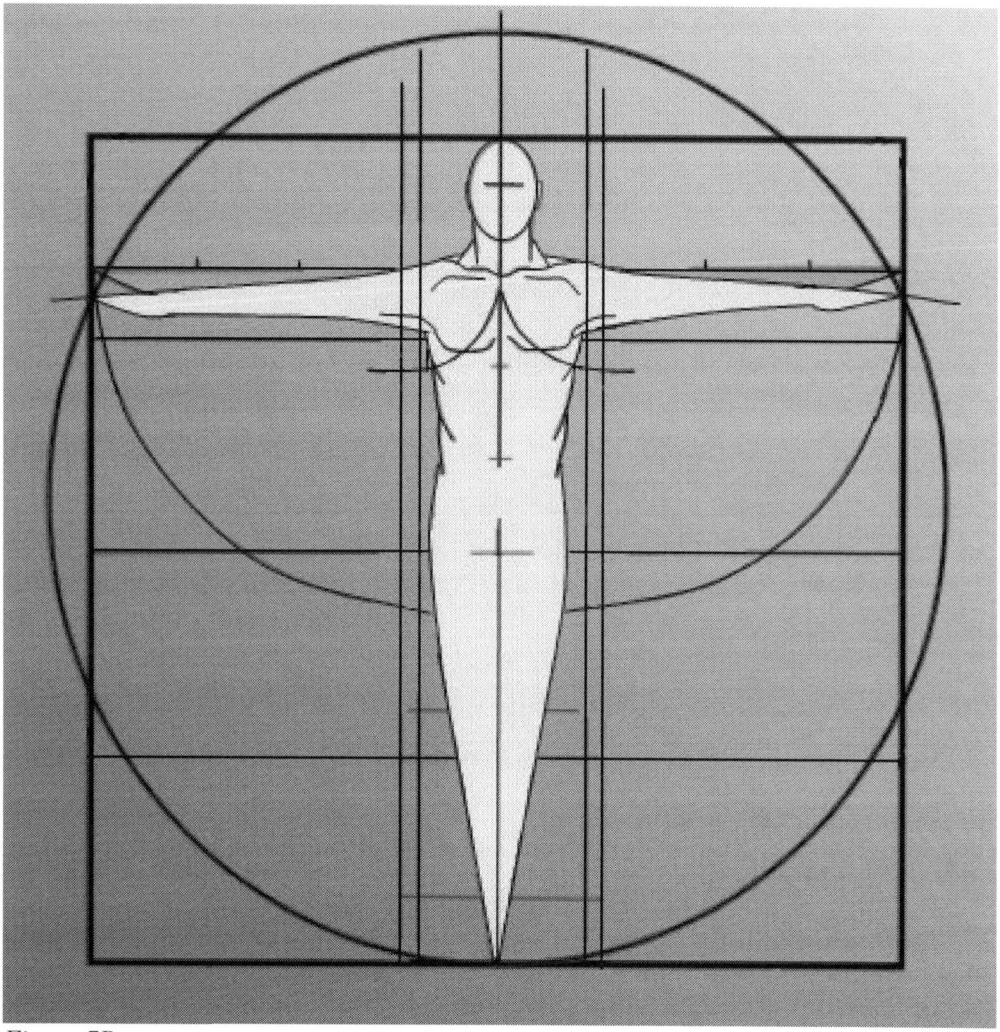

Figure 7B

My Da Vinci Man #3 is basically the same as Leonardo's Vitruvian Man; except I have left the arm rotations and we can find the placement of the knees. The top of the knees are halfway between the navel, at this whole circle, and the bottom of the square. I also made my body form a more delineated version in order to make it easier to find the proportions without the details of the body. Here's my Da Vinci Man #3.

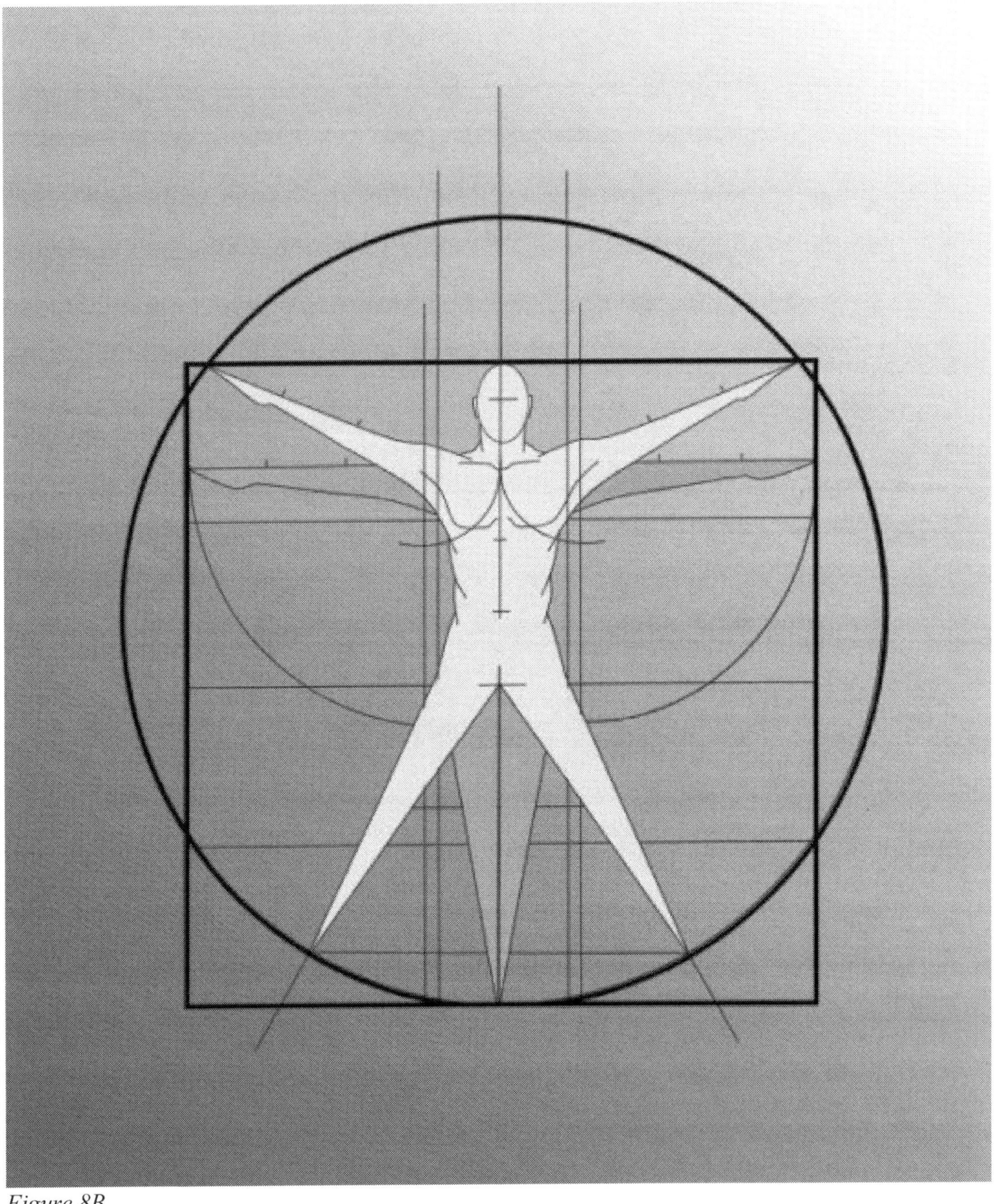

Figure 8B

In the Da Vinci Man #4, we will use Figure 4B and we'll add the inside arm rotation, as seen in Figure 7A. See Figure 9B.

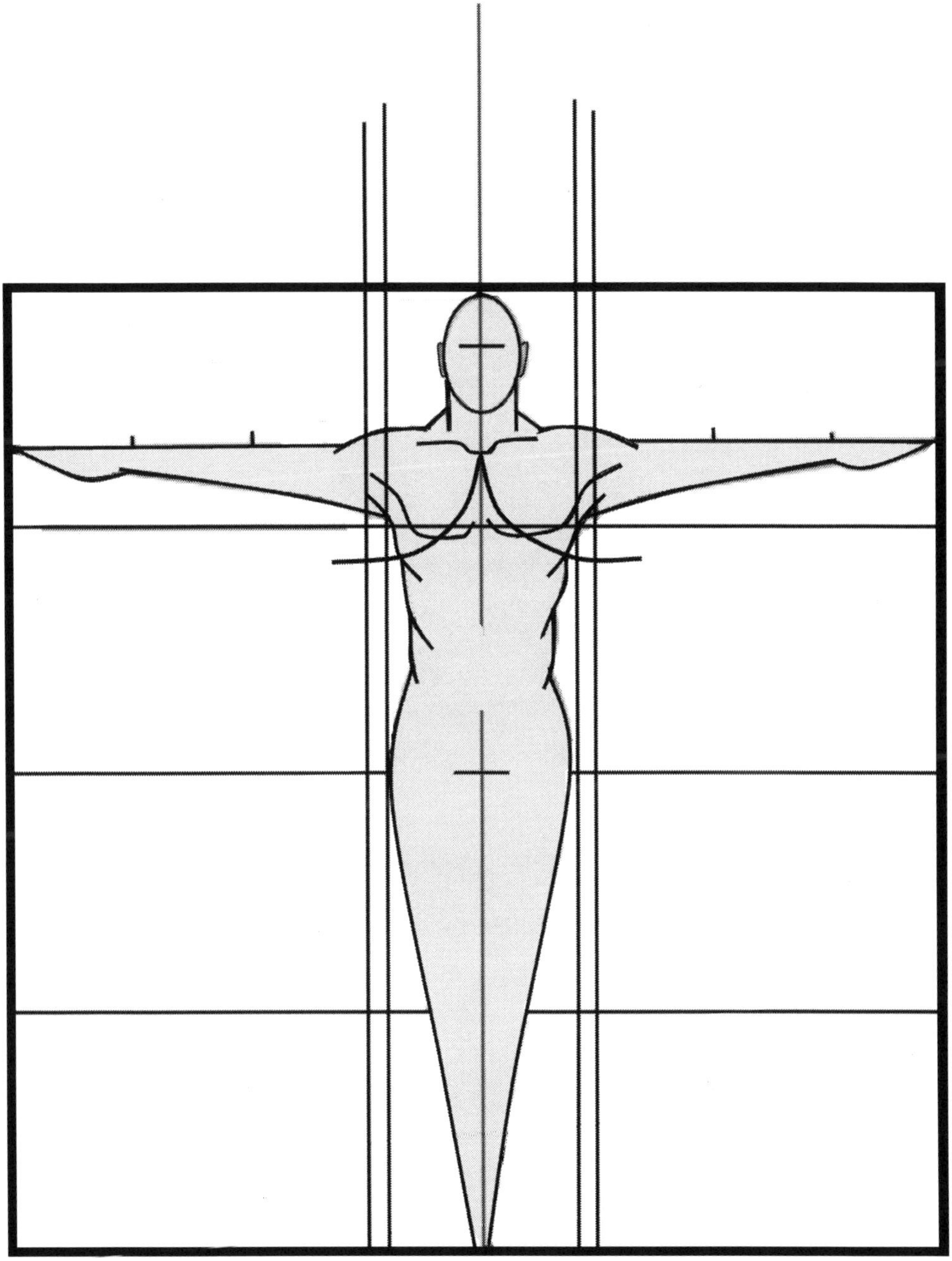

Figure 9B

Draw an upper arm rotation with the point of origin at the 1/5 vertical line and the 1/6 horizontal line, moving the rotation up above the head. See Figure 10B.

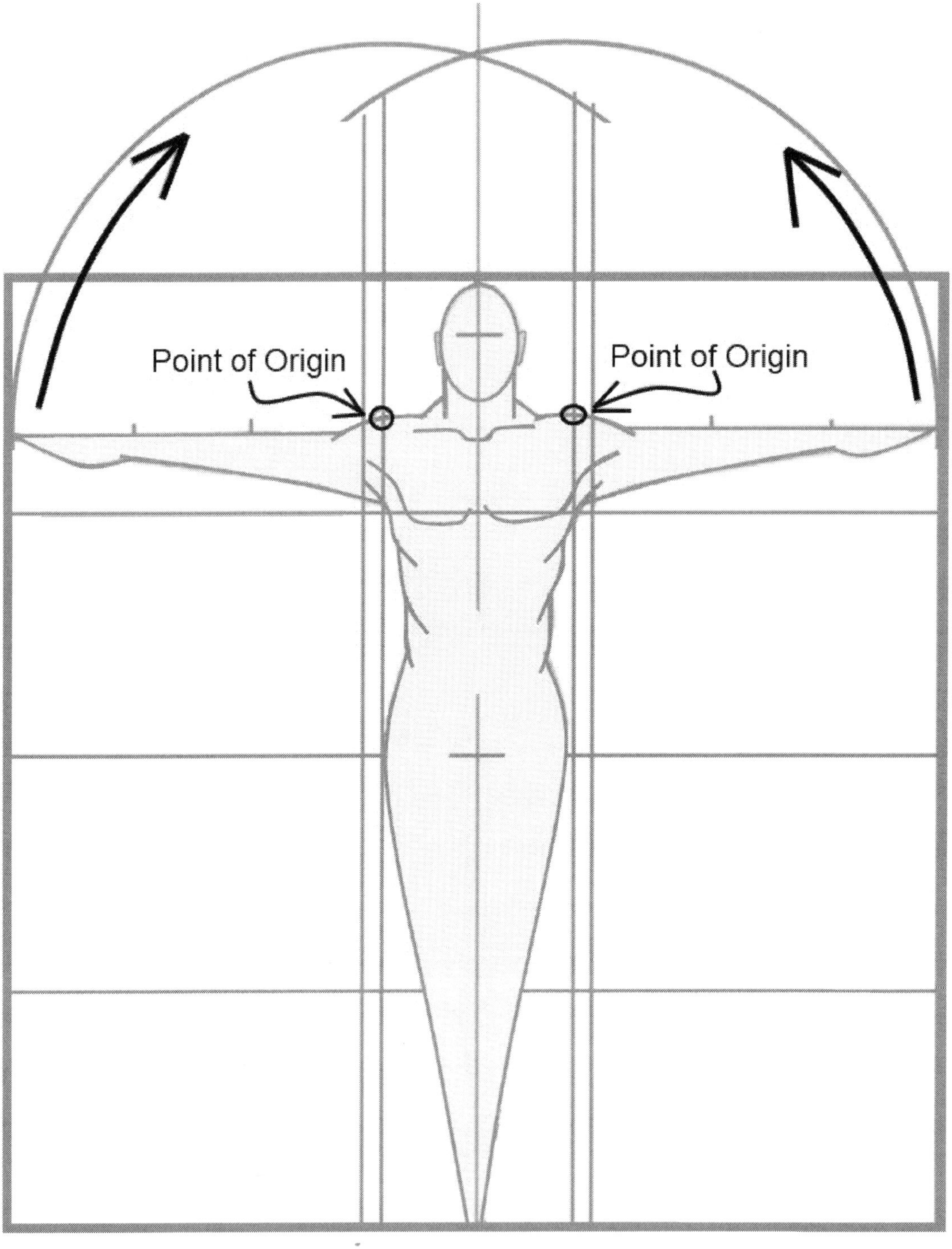

Figure 10B

Now draw an outer whole circle with it stretching approximately ¼ the size of the square above the top of the square. For the 5 inch square this measurement will be 6.25 inches.

The diameter is 6.25 inches and the radius is 3.125 inches. See Figure 11B.

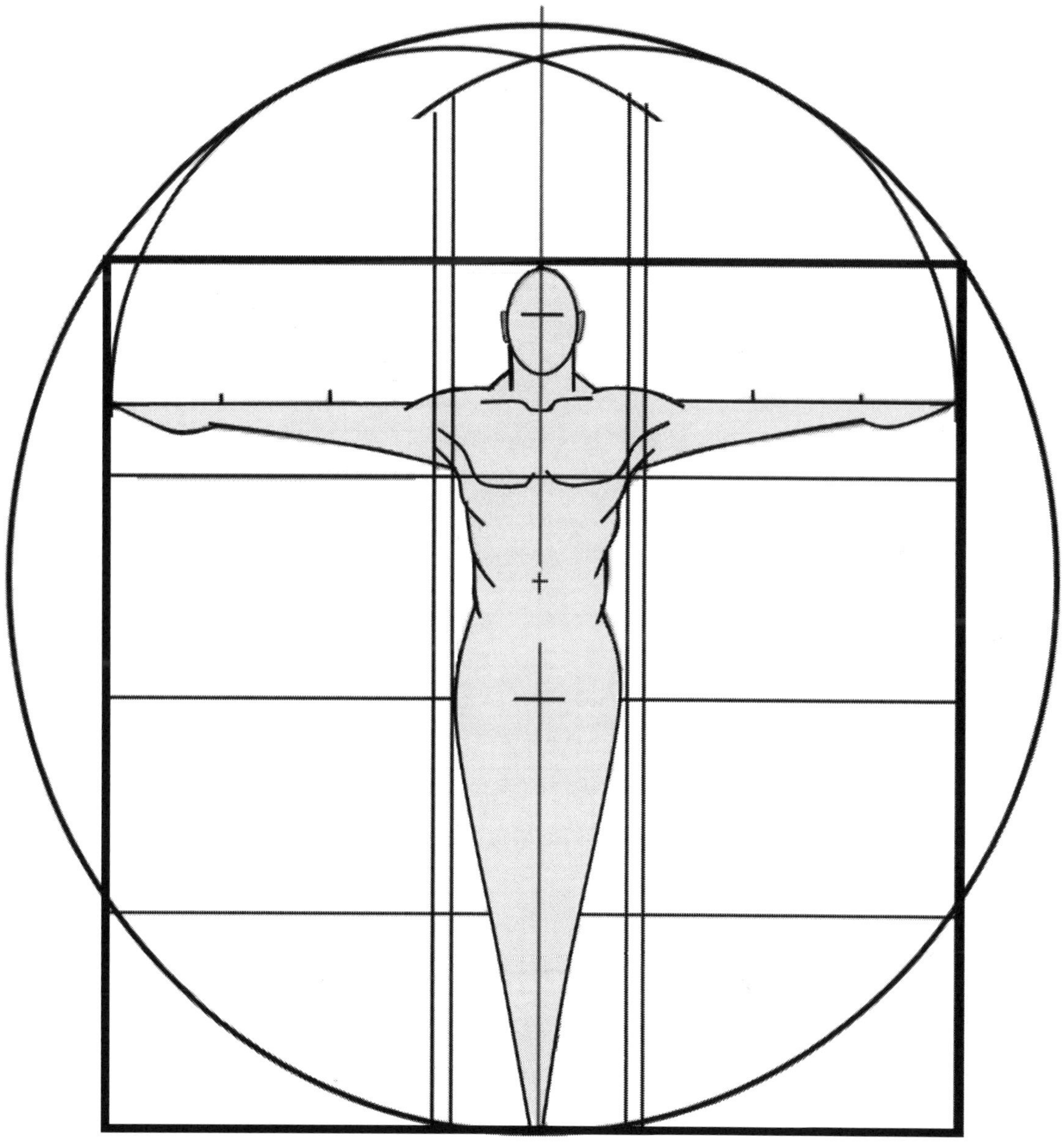

Figure 11B

The arm positions are found by using the ¼ horizontal line from the top of the square and the vertical center line of the square as the origin for the arms. This line will pass through where the outer whole circle touches the upper arm rotation. For a 5 inch square it is 0.77168 inches from the top of the square. Draw a line under the chin of the body's head, this will cross through the 1/5 line at the arm line. See Figure 12B.

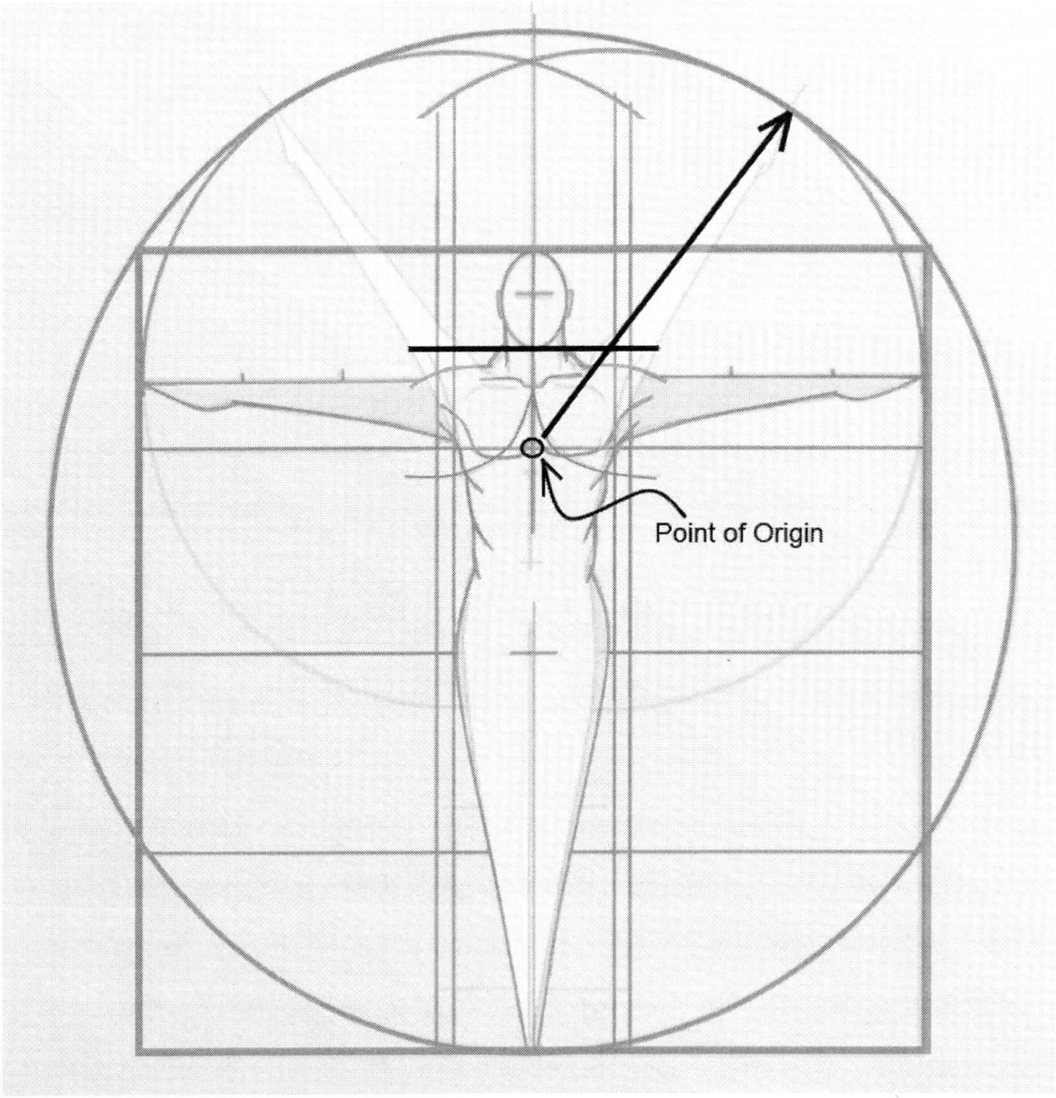

Figure 12B

Since we are dealing with a "floating" joint, I believe at these points the shoulder's point of origin moves from one to another, therefore we have to measure the arm at different locations, depending on which rotation it might be in. This is my Da Vinci Man #4 completed, see Figure 13B.

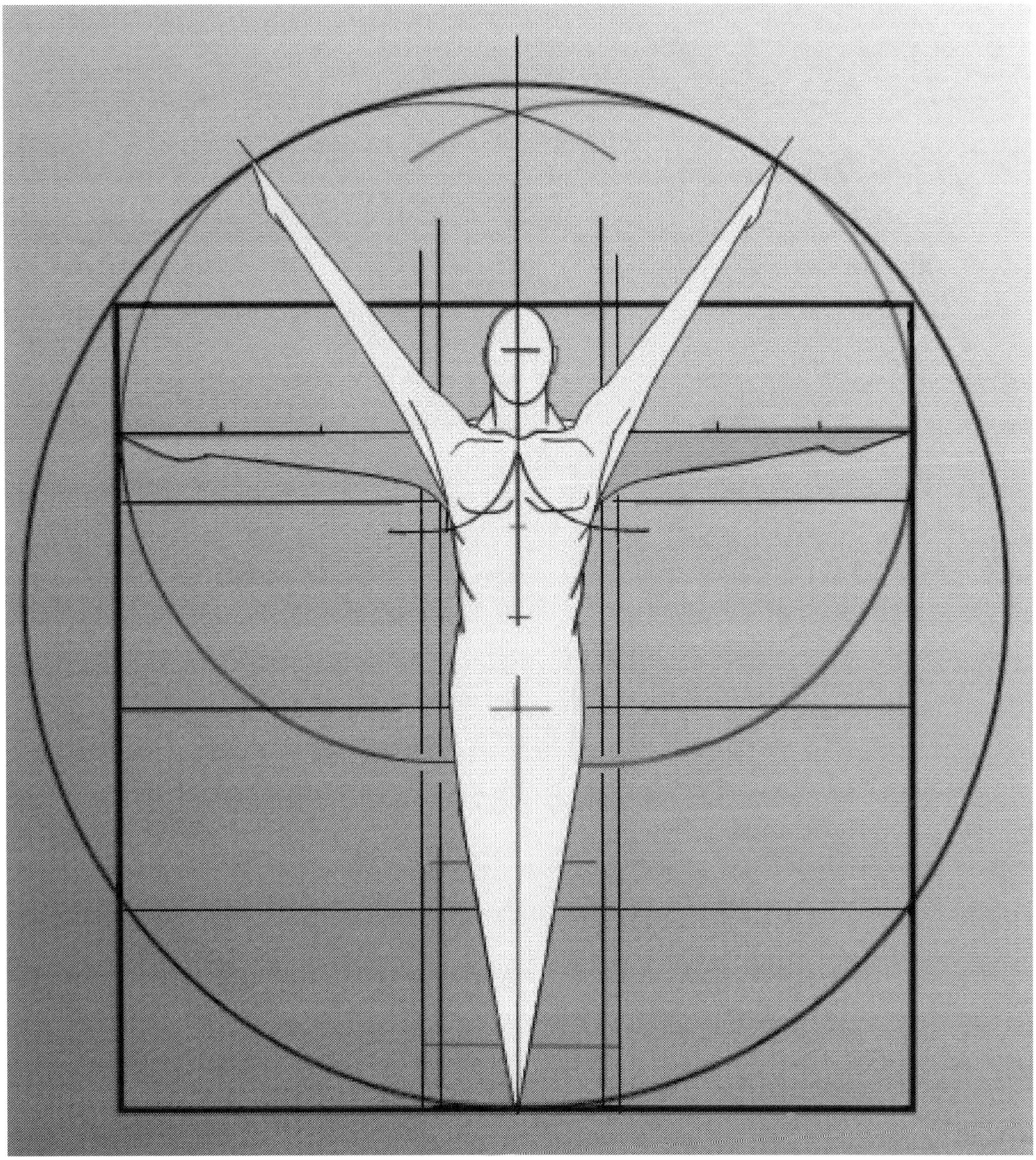

Figure 13B

Now for the final example, Da Vinci Man #5, we will use the design in Figure 10B as a starting point. See Figure 14B.

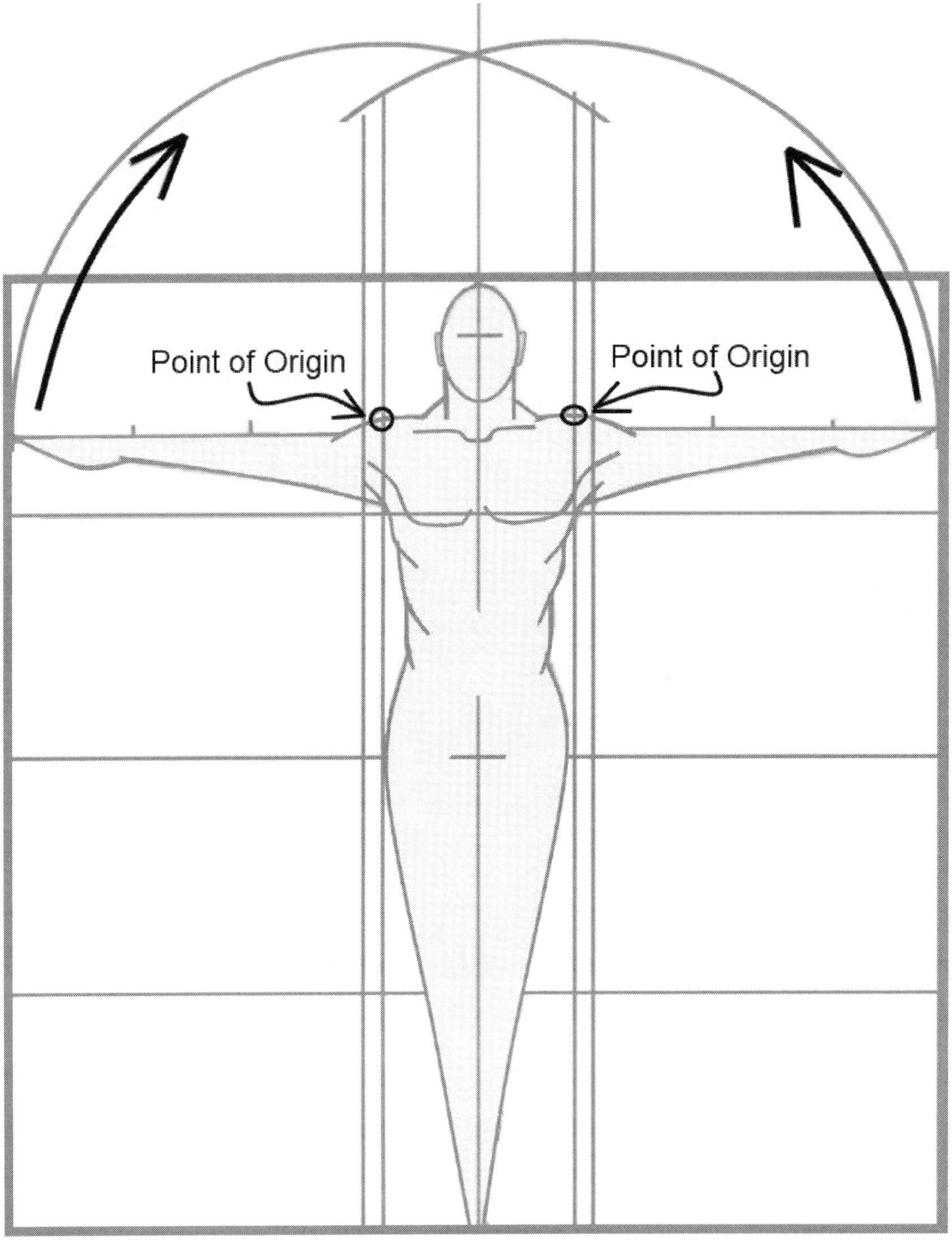

Figure 14B

Draw a line horizontally at 5/8 the body length, just under the chin. Then draw an arc at where the 5/8 line crosses the 1/5 vertical line. The point of origin will be at the center and the 1/6 horizontal line. See Figure 15B.

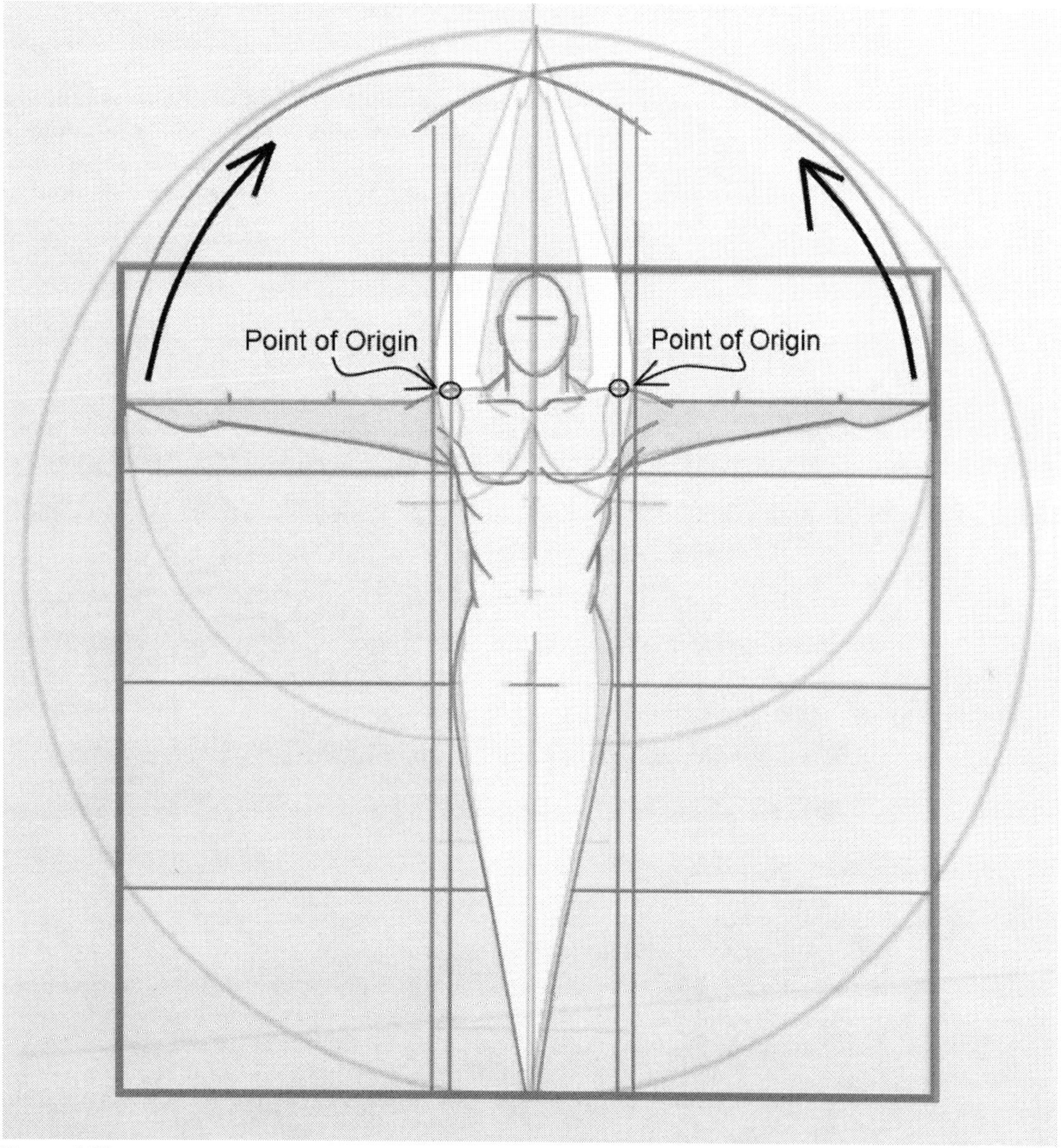

Figure 15B

The rotation arc is the last rotation of the arm in this plane. It begins where the last arm rotation ended in my Da Vinci Man #4 and ends above the head. This last rotation of the arms is an extension of how the arms move within the shoulder; the arms stretch and the shoulder moves up as we reach around, and above our head. This one measurement is where I found myself scratching my own head; I couldn't figure out the best way to solve this problem. That's when I investigated the problem with a few volunteers; the common approximation was that the arms do reach above the point where the last Da Vinci Man left off, but was there also a common ratio to measure with?

The measurement of this circle would begin to take shape at approximately around a ratio of 0.28 between the top of the square and the top edge of the where the circle should be. The floating joint of the shoulder once again proved to be a challenge; but I believe that this measurement is accurate, and later you see why this measurement should be 0.28. The measurement of the arm length will be from the 1/5 vertical line to the edge of the square. Multiply the square by 0.028 to find the measurement for this circle. Now the arm length will be drawn from the point of origin; Figure 15B, to above the head, this will be the top of the circle. See Figure 16B, this is my Da Vinci Man #5.

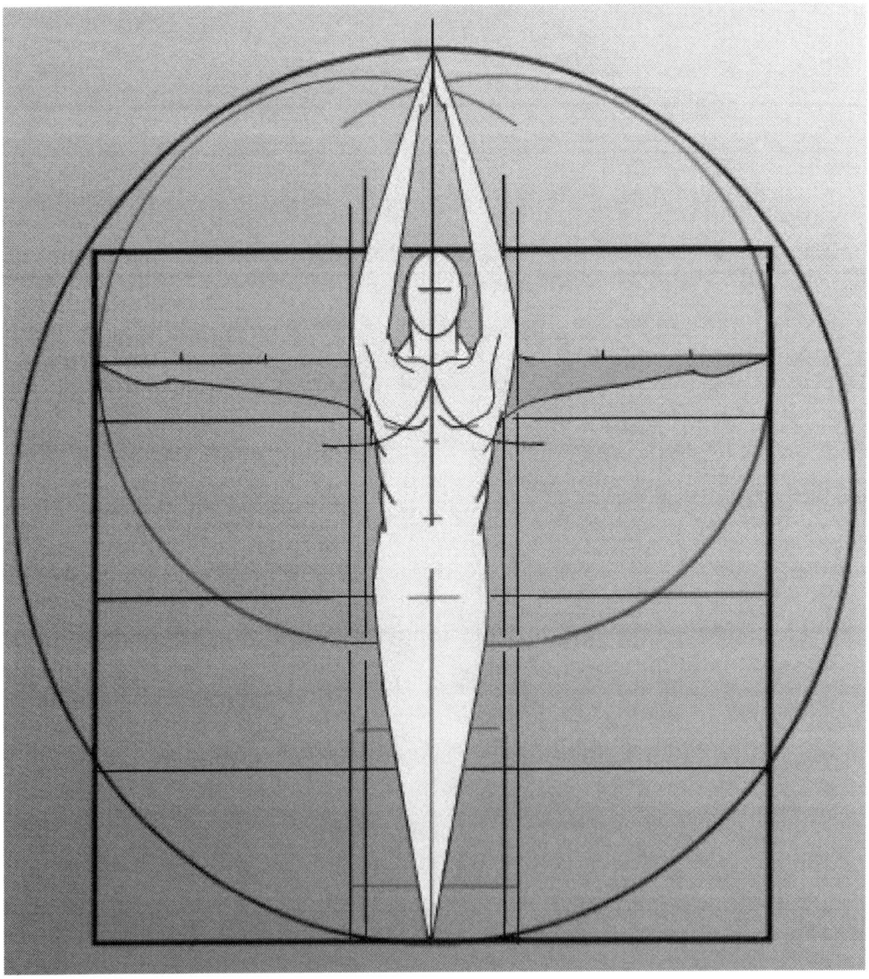

Figure 16B

These four alternative Da Vinci Men may have never graced a final drawing by da Vinci; but in order to find out why there might be some kind of basic form of proportion for the human body, I believe that da Vinci would have applied some kind of math to prove that it could be possible, and he would have wanted to prove to the world that it would be possible. Once he established every form of the body within this set, he would have seen that there is a unique design in the way our arms move within this set.

Let's first describe this set of circles as it relates to the square. The circle must encompass the body and the arm rotation as the hands "push" the circle outwards as the arms move within the arm rotation. In other words, the whole circle must have within itself at all times: the body (from head to toe) and the arms (as they move within their own arm rotation). The circle cannot be smaller than the height of the body, nor can the circle be larger than the outstretched arms above the head, therefore we can state one rule of the set.

The restricted set of circles must remain tangent to the square where the vertical center line crosses the square side and the circle, the feet of the body anchor the circle to the square, but can also move within this set. This would be a point to which da Vinci would have seen before anyone else; it can be seen in the way his drawing has the man with a beginning form with the feet anchored to the bottom center. If he thought that this one piece of information wasn't important; then would he have even had the man begin at this position? He knew that it needed to start here, because with every human body our feet will always anchor us to nature. See Figure 17B.

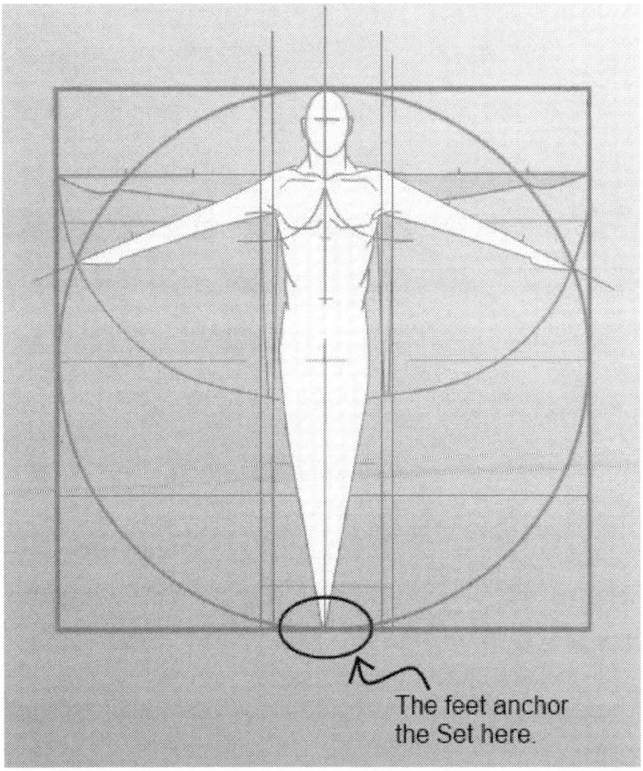

Figure 17B

When we begin to see how the circle increases in diameter beyond the constraints of the square, we find that a proportional variable arises. See Figure 18B.

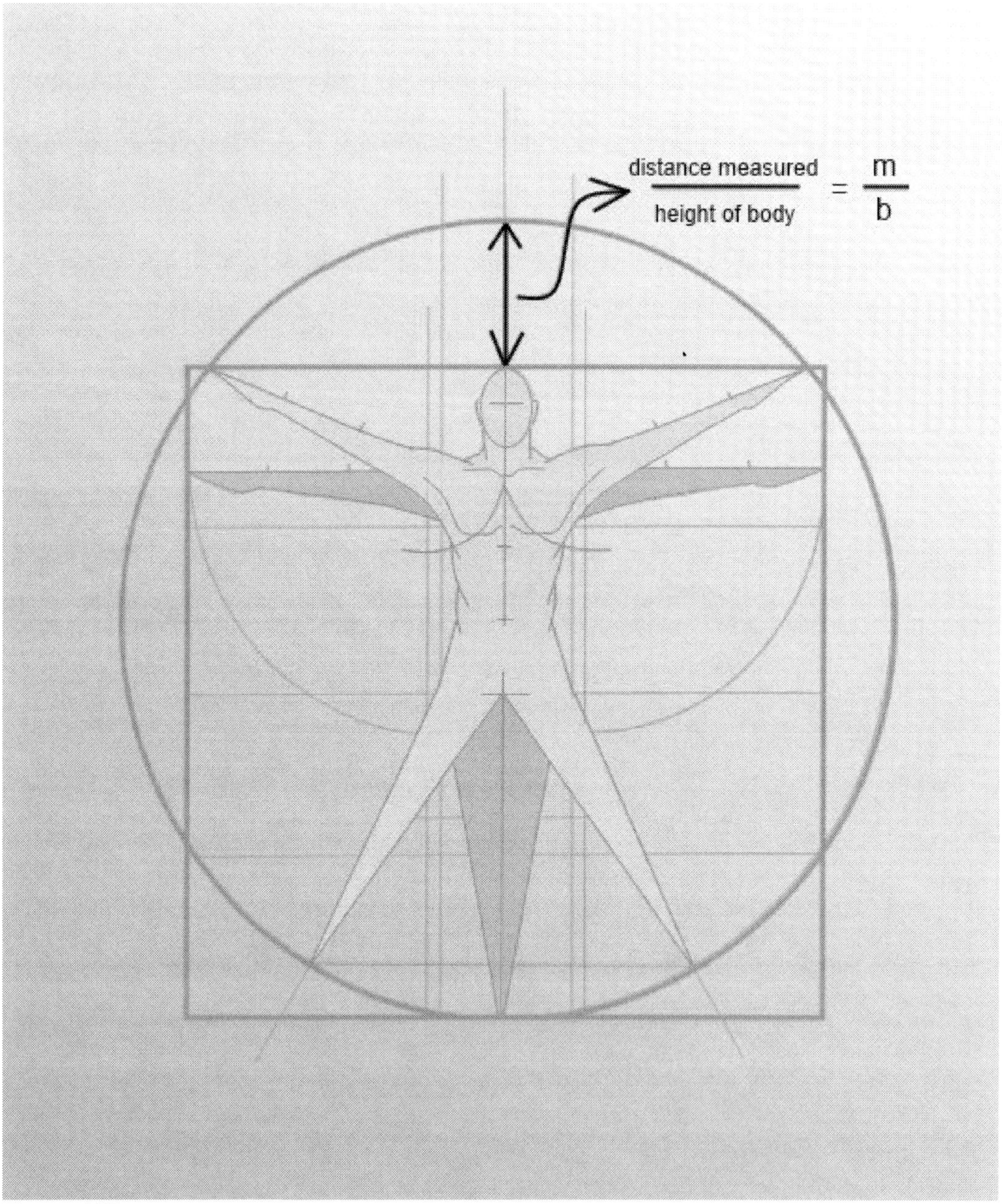

Figure 18B

As we can see in Figure18B, when we divide the distance between the circle and the square (m) by the height of the square (b), then we define a proportional variable (k), therefore: $m/b = k$, when $b>0$, $k \geq 0$.

To find the diameter of the circle, we need to multiply the height of the body or the square (b) by the proportional variable (k), then add it to the height of the body or the square (b), therefore we can say: $kb + b = d$.

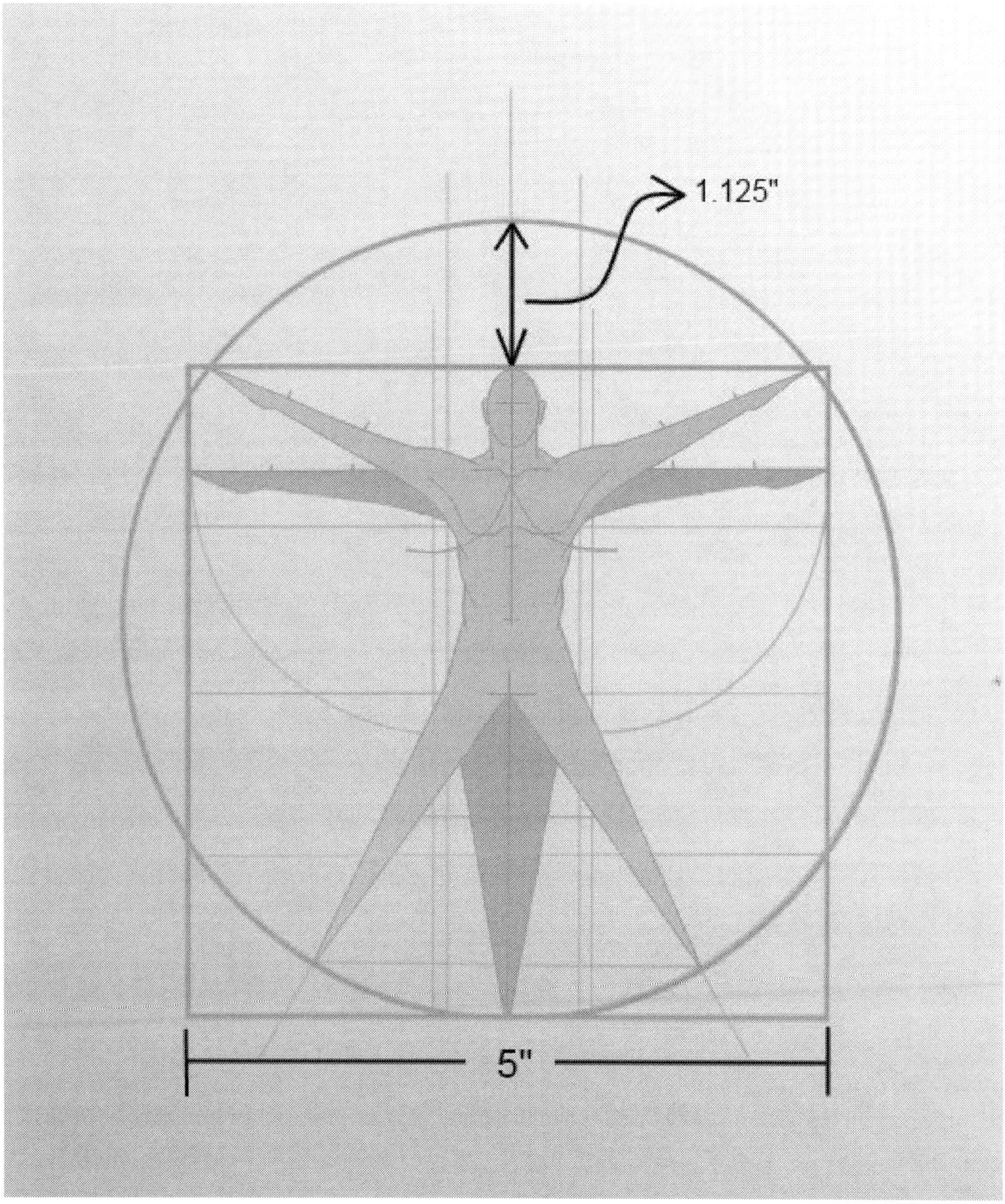

Figure 19B

When $k = 1.125/5 = 0.225$ then, $kb+b=d$; $d = (0.225)5 + 5 = 6.125$"

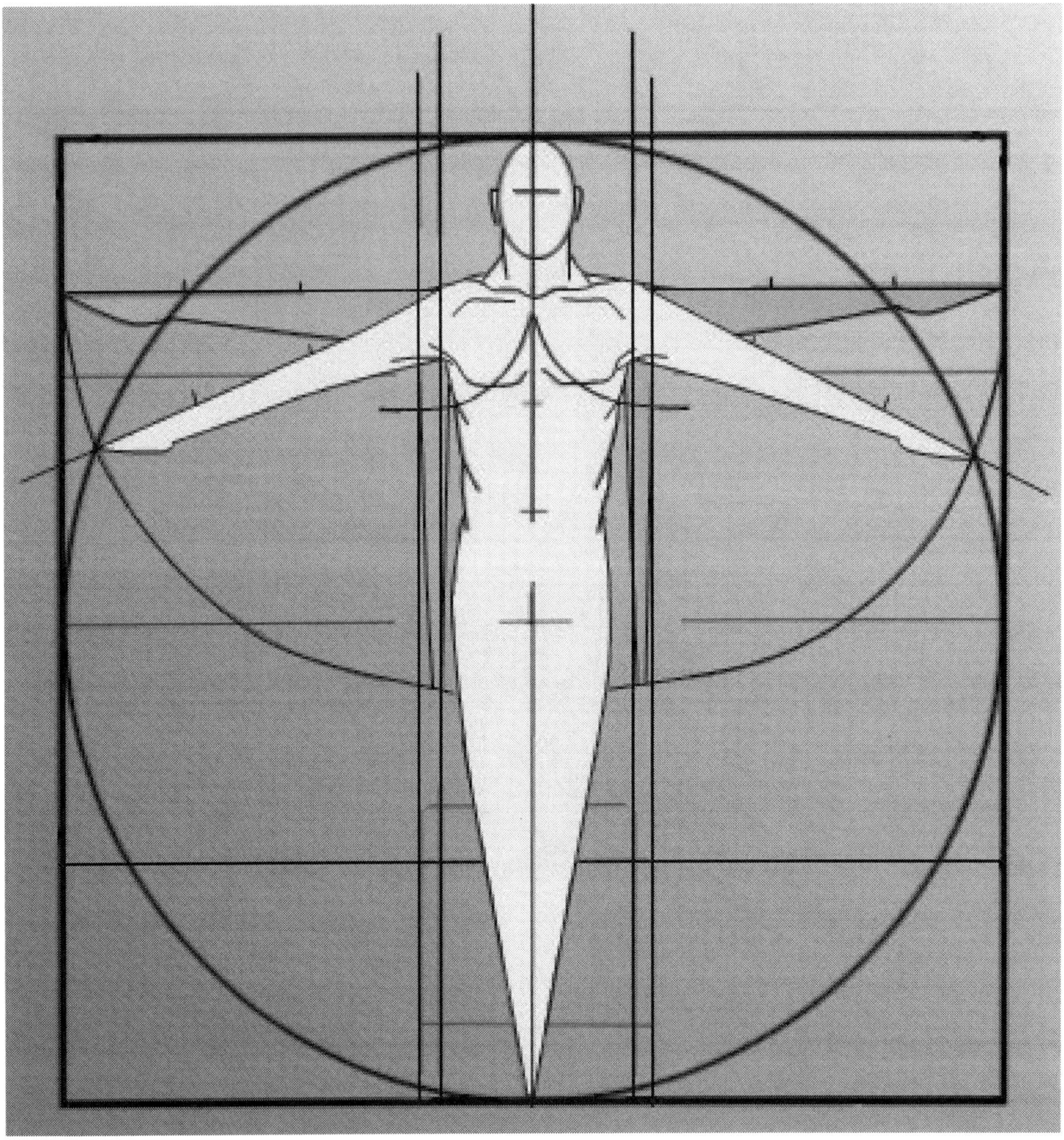

Figure 20B

When the proportional variable is at k = 0, the circle and the square center are both at the same position. Since this "set of circles" are restricted, we must define that restriction as: $0 \leq k \leq 0.28$. This is another key component that can't be overlooked. This is where we began are set of Da Vinci Men.

At k = 0.28 (Da Vinci Man #5), we need to make a few measurements to better compare it to the rest of the Da Vinci Men. Look at Figure 21B.

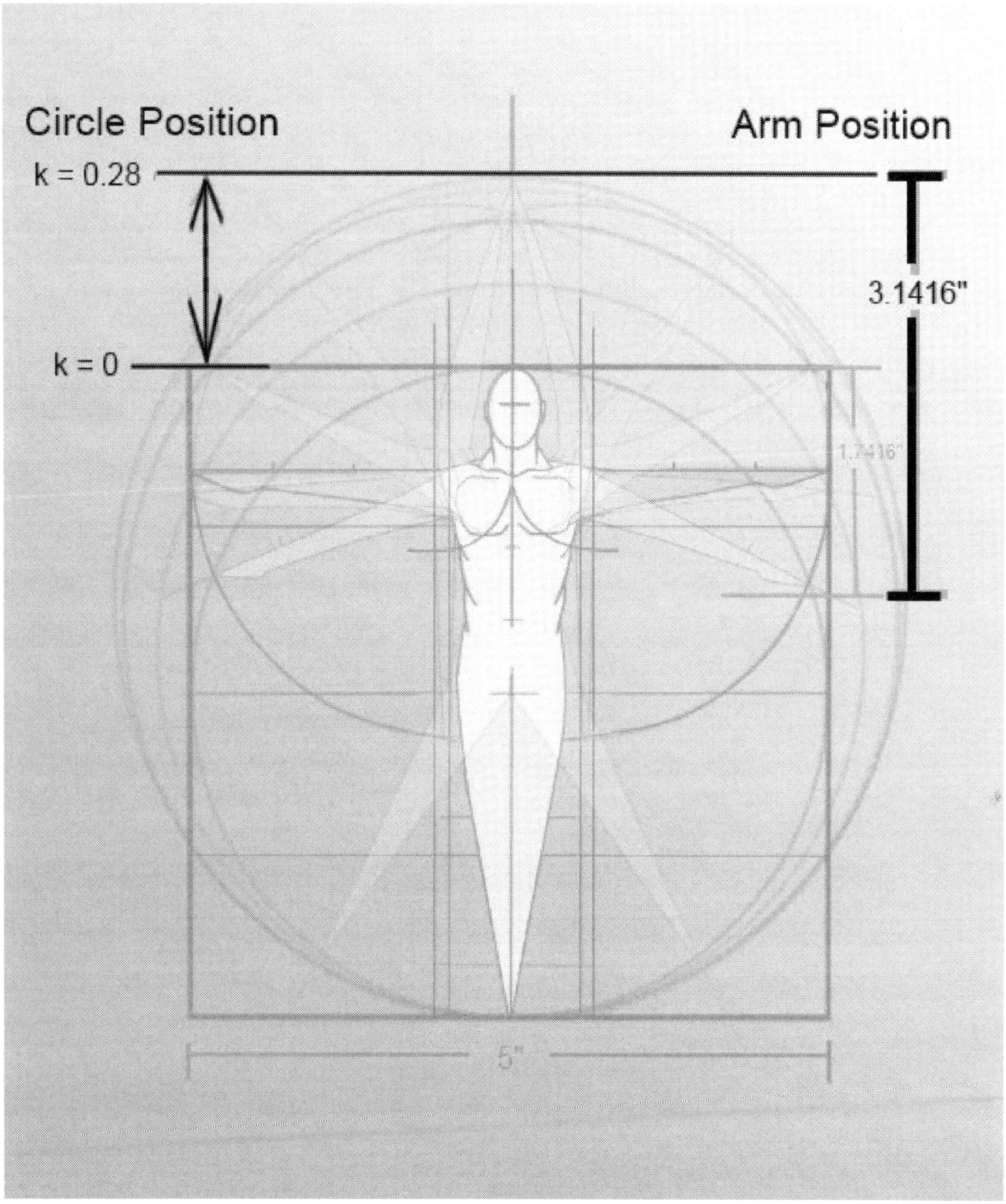

Figure 21B

You may notice that the measurement of the arm position range, from k = 0 to k = 0.28, is a rounded version of pi (π). This feature is very important. This is only a measurement, but if we relate it to the square, then we can find a proportional constant between the arm positions and the square. The one measurement we are concerned with right now will be the distance from the top of the square to the hand position at k=0, the distance I am referring to is 1.7416" on Figure 21B. This distance will remain proportional to the square always, so therefore we can make a proportional constant by dividing it by the square: 1.7416/5 = 0.34832.

If we want to find the distance left between the hand position and the bottom of the square, then we can say: b – (0.34832)b = 5 – 1.7416 = 3.2584". We'll call this distance q. Now to verify the measurement of 3.1416", we say: diameter of the k = 0.28 circle minus what we call q. Example: d#5 + (0.28)b + b = 6.4"; q = 3.2584"; then d#5 – q = 6.4 – 3.2584 = 3.1416". Let's call this distance p, and then relate it to the square by p/b = 3.1416/5 = 0.62832. This is another proportional constant in this set of circles.

This is a secret to understanding the set of Da Vinci Men. This constant is the distance between the navel or the center of the circle and the top of the circle, always. Therefore making itself a constant, it remains the same throughout the total movement of the mechanism. It's the backbone of the whole mechanism, it holds the three (body, square, and circle) together as a whole set.

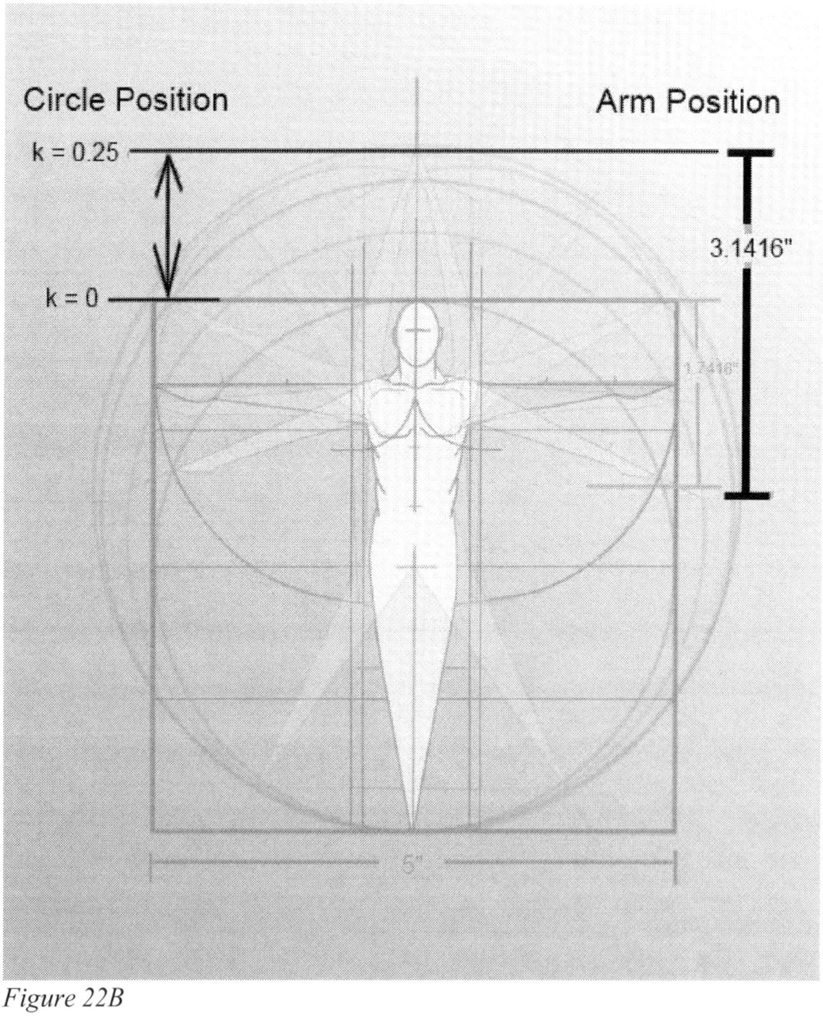

Figure 22B

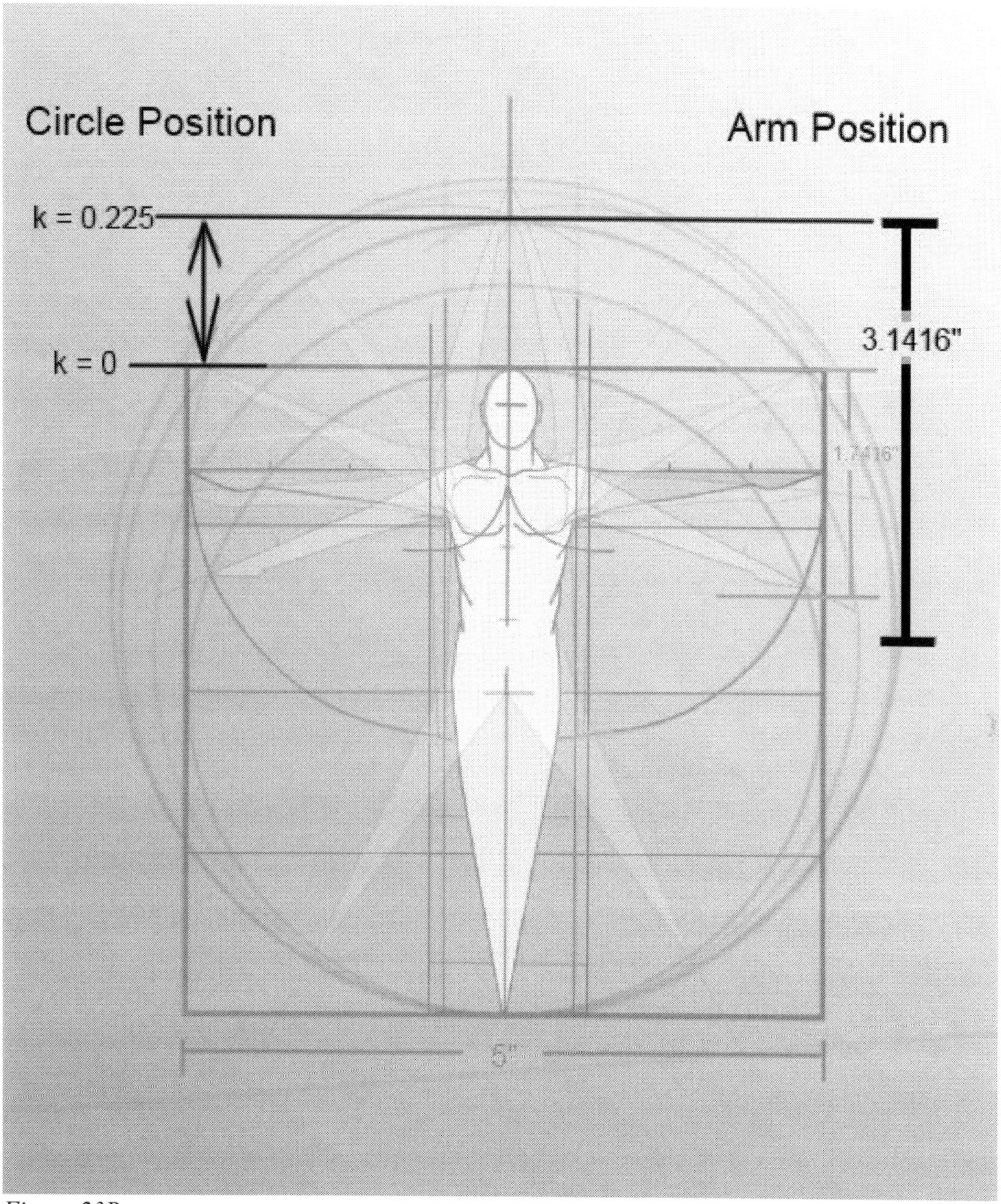

Figure 23B

As the arm position moves down, the mechanism will follow. Notice how the measurement of 3.1416" seems to follow the same way the mechanism works.

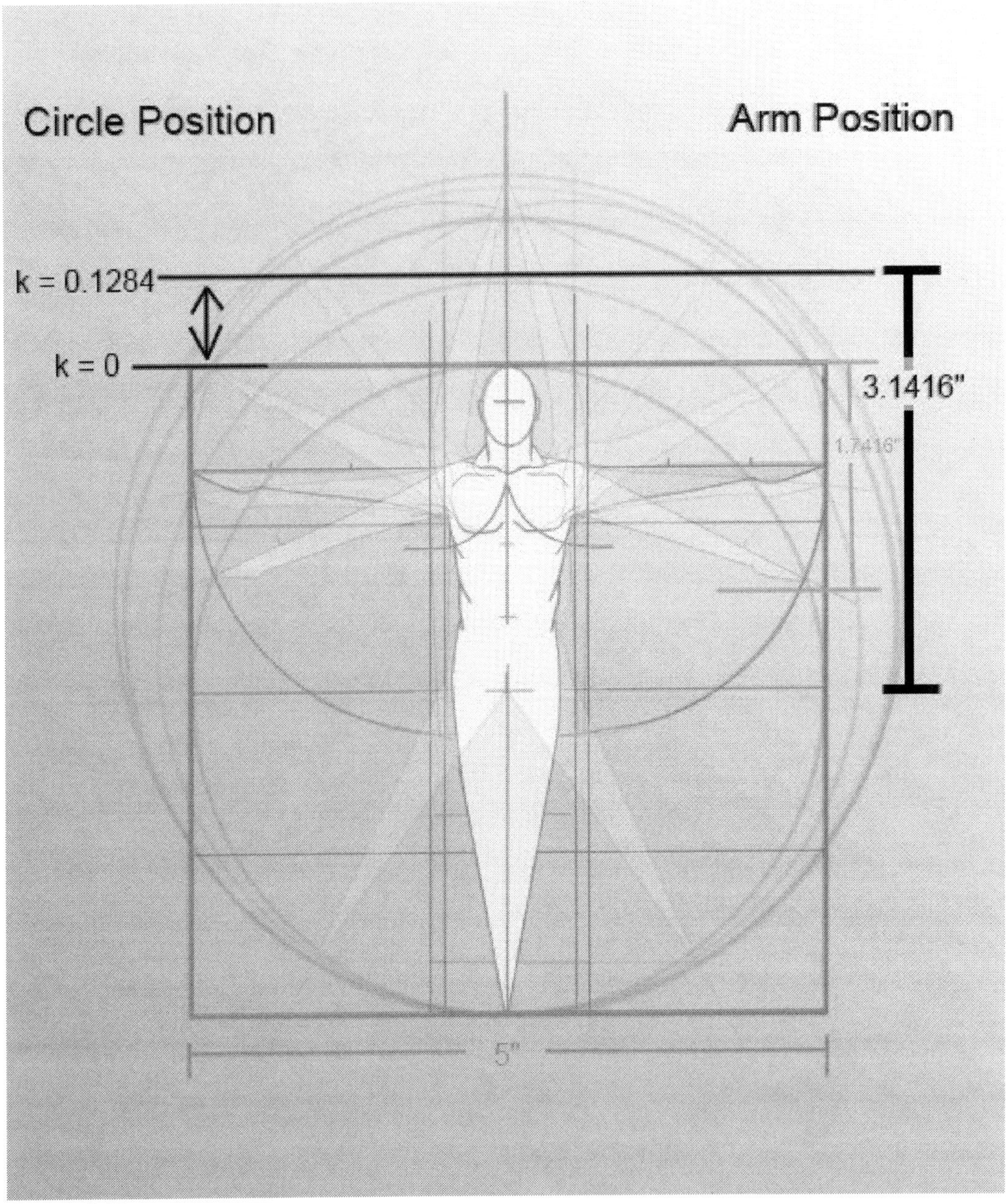

Figure 24B

At this position, the circle and the square area is most equal, notice where the bottom of the mechanism is; it's on the square's center line.

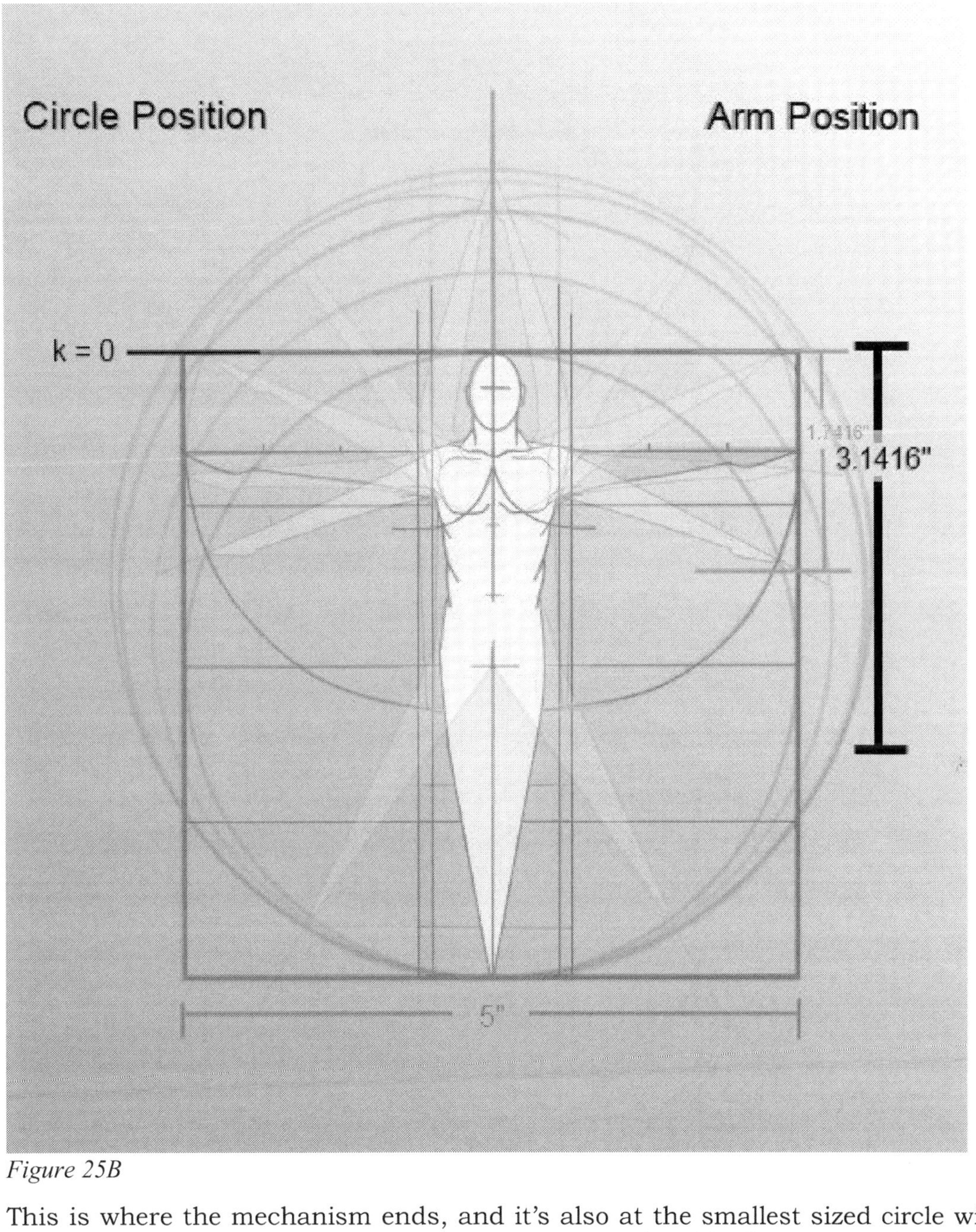

Figure 25B

This is where the mechanism ends, and it's also at the smallest sized circle within the set of circles. When the arm positions are measured inside the square, the lines are to be straight until they reach the side of the square, but when the arm position is measured above the square; where they meet the circle, is where they are to be measured to.

At a 2 inch diameter, or 1 inch radius, the area for a circle is exactly pi (π) and the area for a square is exactly 4. The ratio between the two will be π/4 or 0.7854. Here's an example:

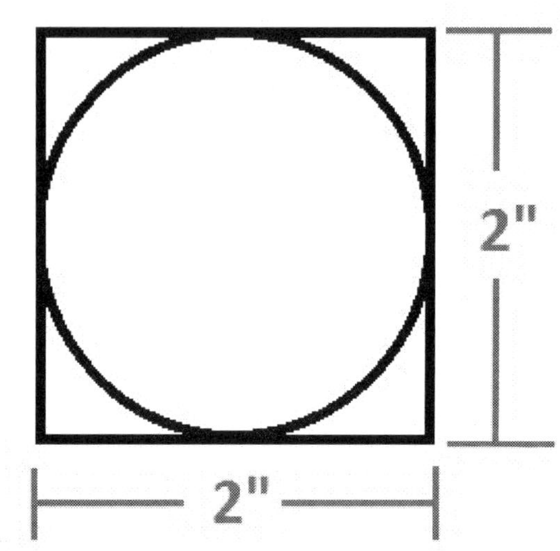

Figure 26B

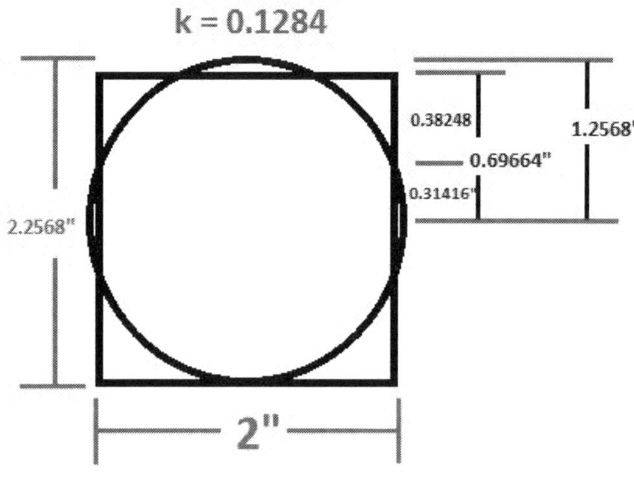

Figure 27B

In Figure 27B we can see how the ratio 0.7854 is represented in a basic form, but if make the circle larger and stay within our set at k = 0.1284, then we can now see the mechanism in its most basic form. Notice the constant, at this measurement, is now measured at 0.31416". The mechanism at any size will stay the same, but of course the circle is dependent on the square.

To find the center of the circle placement, measuring from the pubis, use the proportional constant from the diameter equation (k), multiply by the length of the square or the height of the body, and then divide it by 2. Here's an example: kb/2 = center of circle placement. Then measure up from the pubis by that number to find the center of circle placement. Here is a chart of the different center of circle placements for a 2 inch square.

Whole Circle	Radius	Navel Placement from Pubis
2.56"	1.28"	0.28"
2.5"	1.25"	0.25"
2.45"	1.225"	0.225"
2.2568"	1.1284"	0.1284"
2"	1"	0

Figure 28B

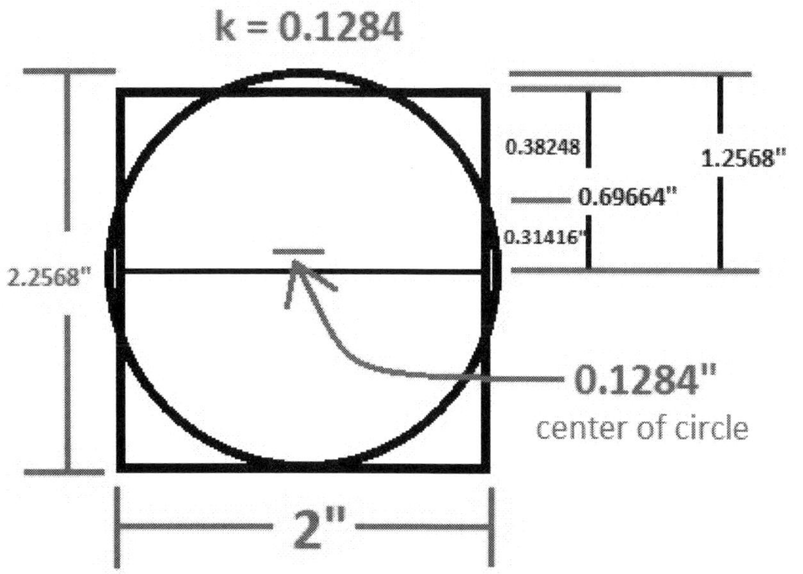

Figure 29B

In Figure 29B, we can see where the center of the circle should go, but it should be noted that it's easier to just find the diameter of the circle and then just divide that by 2, than to use this method. So why did I even bring it up? It's to show how that, as the magnitude of the circle increases, so too will the center move up from the pubic region in a correlated manner. When the center of the circle reaches the natural center of gravity; as da Vinci will have you believe, the center will then represent the position of the navel. To find that position we merely use a simple equation such as, the diameter of the Vitruvian Man circle divided by two, or we could say, dV/2 = navel placement.

Since da Vinci was so obsessed with squaring the circle; an impossible solution to really solve, I've created a simple solution that could have been looked at by him, and it incorporates the set of Da Vinci Men.

Use a compass to draw a large circle, large enough to outline the square you want to draw.

Use the edge of the circle as a point of origin, and then draw an arc that passes through the center as seen in Figure 30B.

Draw a line through the two points where the arc passes through the circle as in Figure 31B.

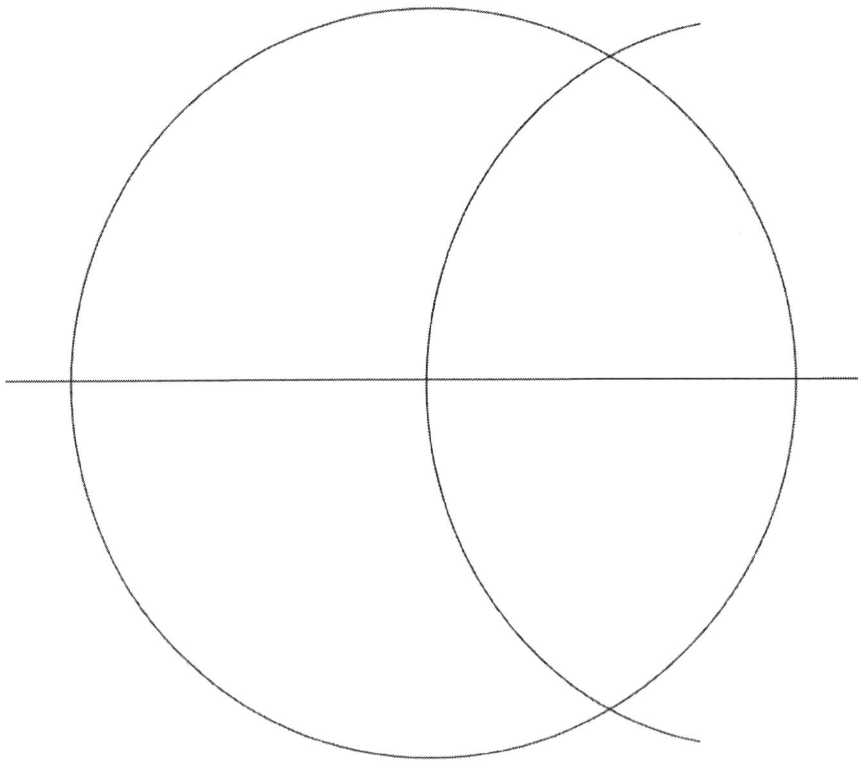

Figure 30B

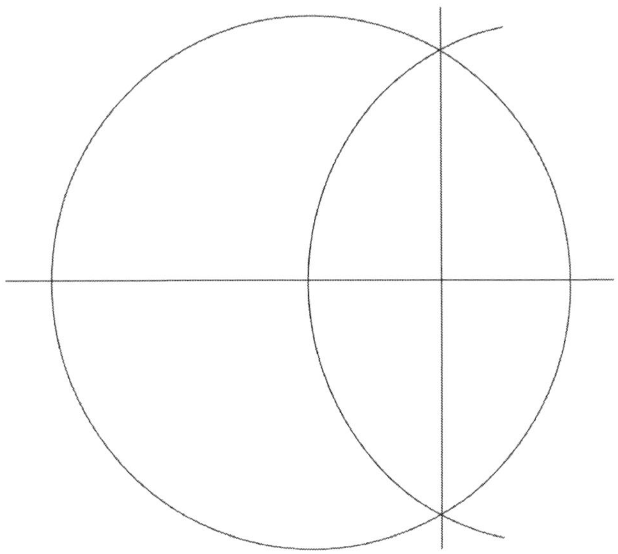

Figure 31B

Use the intersection of the line that passes through the arc and circle as a point of origin for a smaller arc that also passes through the center and the line as seen in Figure 32B.

Draw a line through the intersection of the smaller arc and the line, through the center of the circle, and pass through the other side of the circle as seen in Figure 33B.

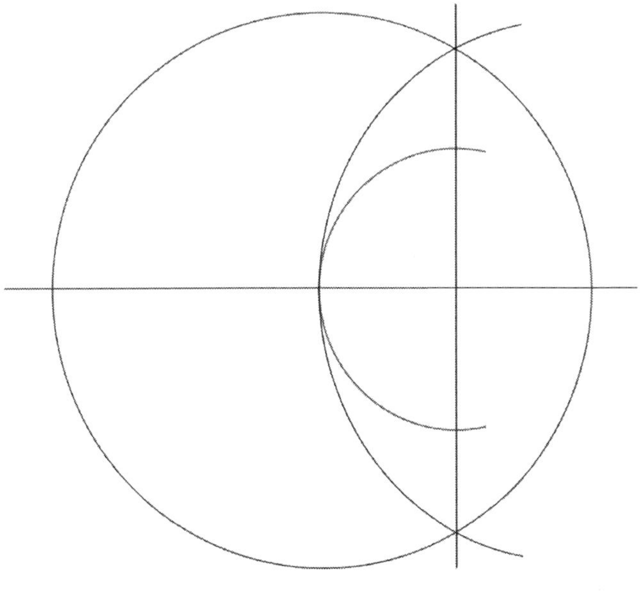

Figure 32B

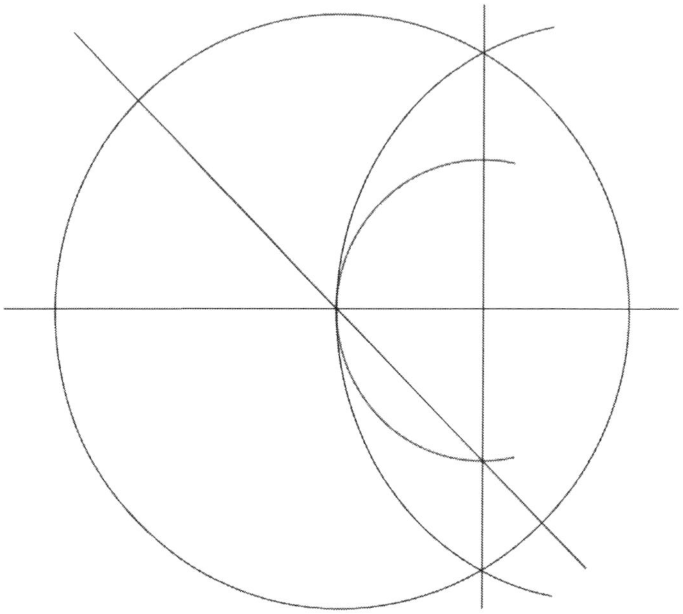

Figure 33B

Draw the other line perpendicular to it as seen in Figure 34B.

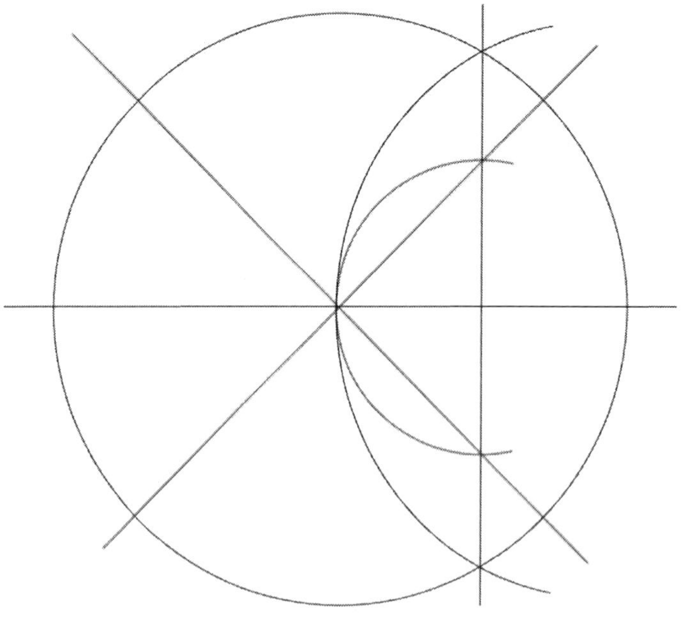

Figure 34B

Draw four lines to connect the four points on the circle as seen in Figure 35B.

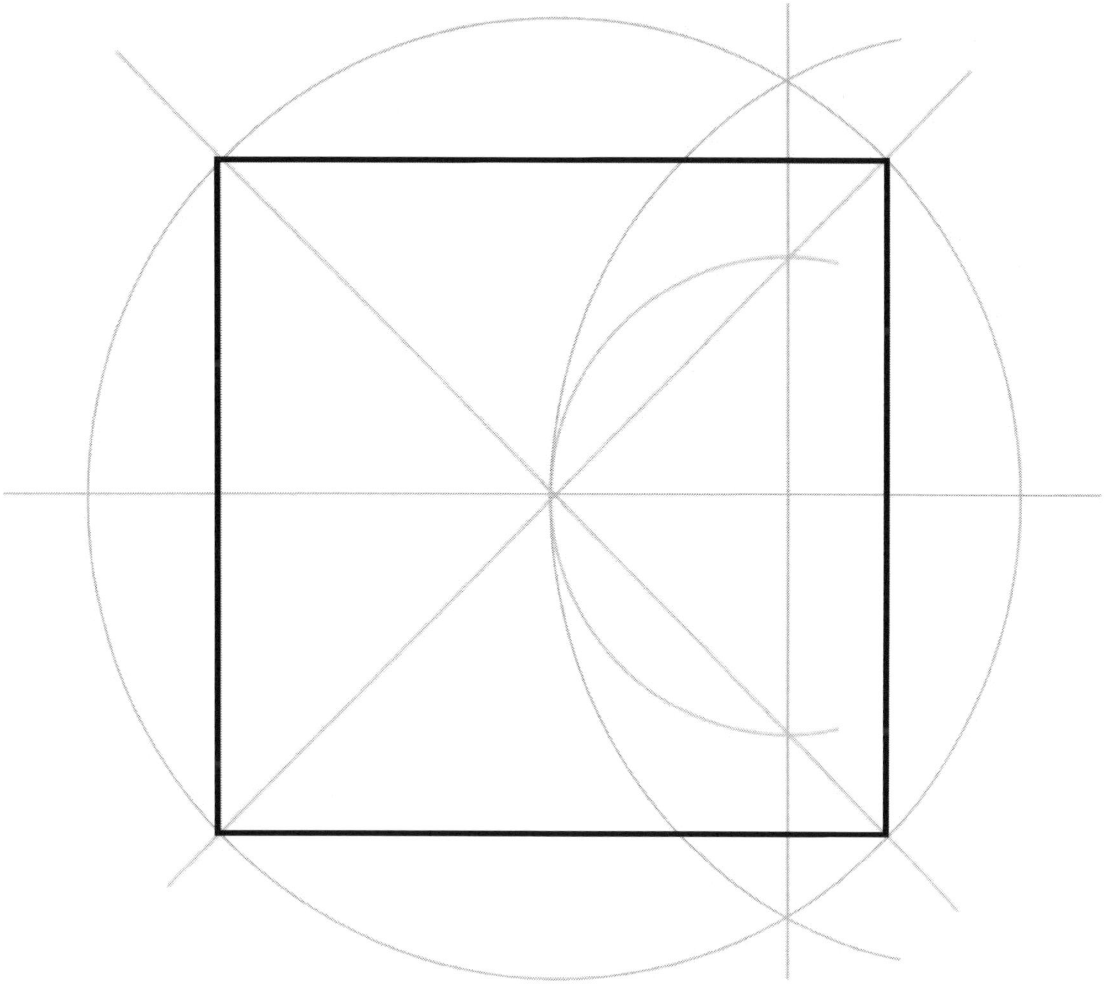

Figure 35B

Erase all the lines that do not make a square, except the line through the center horizontally, as seen in Figure 36B.

Divide the top half of the square in two equal distances. Lay the straightedge along the line, estimate where the half mark should go and mark that spot, on the paper as well as the straightedge, as seen in Figure 37B.

Figure 36B

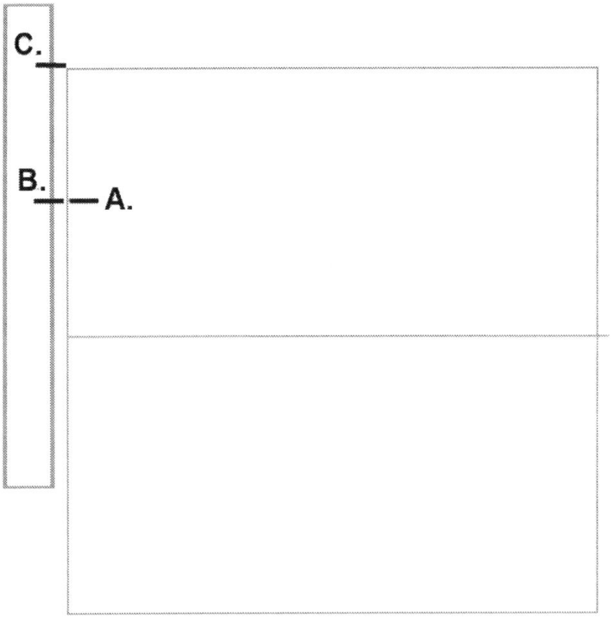

Figure 37B

Check it by measuring the two halves with the mark on the straightedge, as seen in Figure 38B. Draw that line as in Figure 39B.

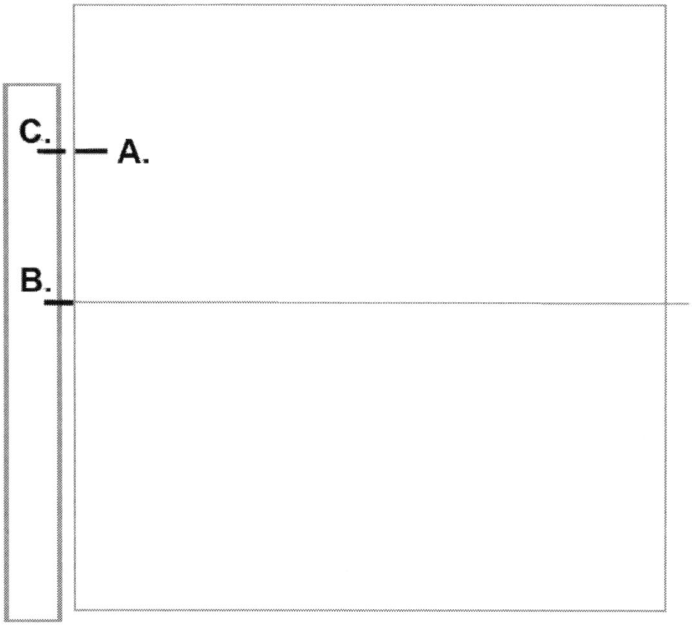

Figure 38B

Figure 39B

Divide the top ¼ of the square in half, same method as above, as seen in Figure 40B.

Use the measurement from Figure 40B to measure above the square the same distance, as seen in Figure 41B.

Figure 40B

Figure 41B

This will give you the diameter of the circle to be drawn tangent to the bottom of the square, as seen in Figure 42B.

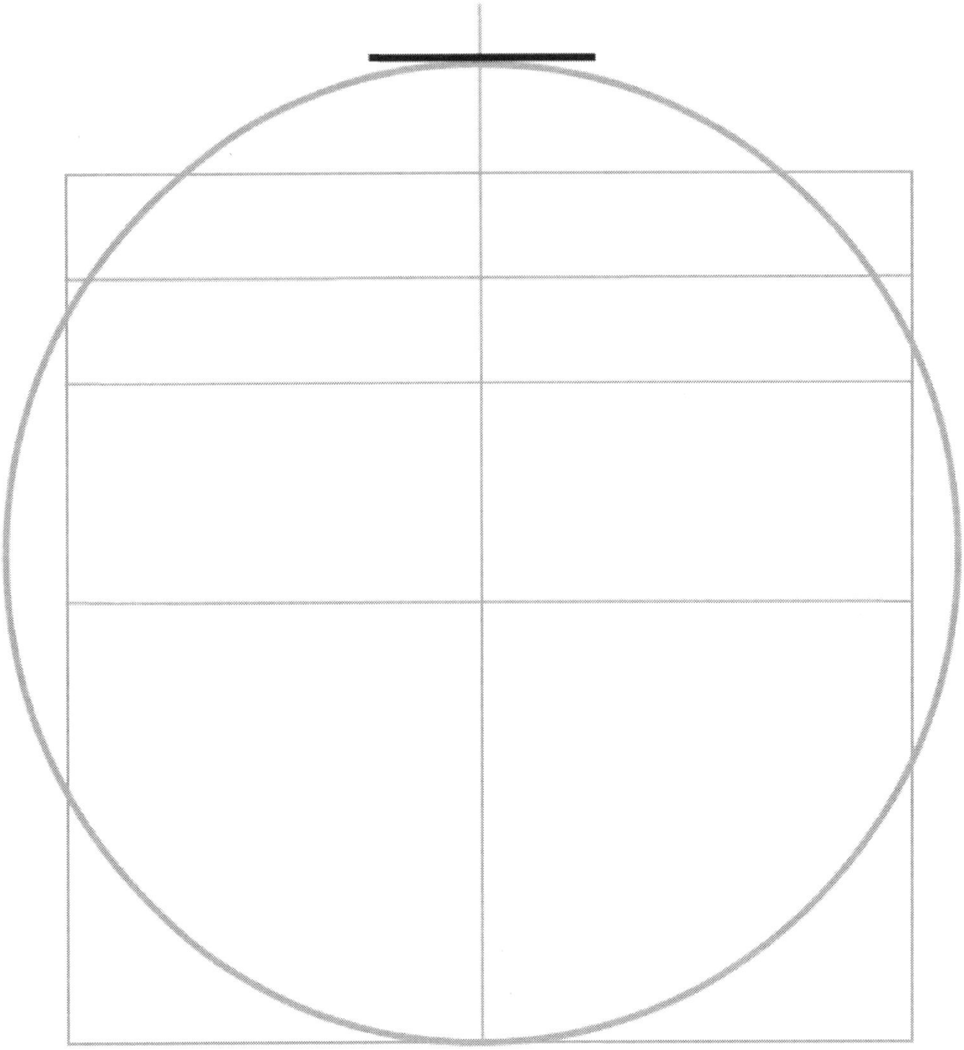

Figure 42B

This will be a close equilibrium between that circle and that square, or at least close enough for just a straightedge and a compass in less than 15 steps. The example I used was measured after it drawn to see how close the two areas are, but before we look at the results, remember that we will use k=0.1284 as the average for 1/8, which is 0.125, because the difference is less than a pencil mark.

a. The area of the square: A ≈ d^2   A ≈ (2.828) ^ 2 ≈ 7.997584
b. The area of the circle: A ≈ πr^2   A ≈ (3.1416)(1.5955576)^2 ≈ 7.9978978

c. The diameter of the circle: $d \approx (0.1284)b + b$

$$d \approx (0.1284)2.828 + 2.828 \approx 3.1911152$$

That's a difference of approximately 0.0003138. I would say that's not bad for a straightedge and a compass.

He could have tried his hand at this solution; it not only incorporates the way we found the different drawings of my Da Vinci Men, but it's also an exploration with geometric implications that were familiar to him at that time. You can see in his notes how he would work with different variations of many different geometric shapes; so it wouldn't be a farfetched idea that he may have explored this solution also.

The Design of the Body

It wasn't only just the idea of trying to prove that a human body could be defined by a simple geometric design that would engross the mind of da Vinci; he would also try to prove how these shapes could be used to describe the human form as a structure of nature. It would be his compulsive character to want to know how the human body worked; to him it was one of the greatest machines ever made by nature. As an artist, he would say that in order to capture the true character of the subject represented in a painting; the artist would have to know everything about that subject, inside and out. This would lead him to the anatomical studies of the human body.

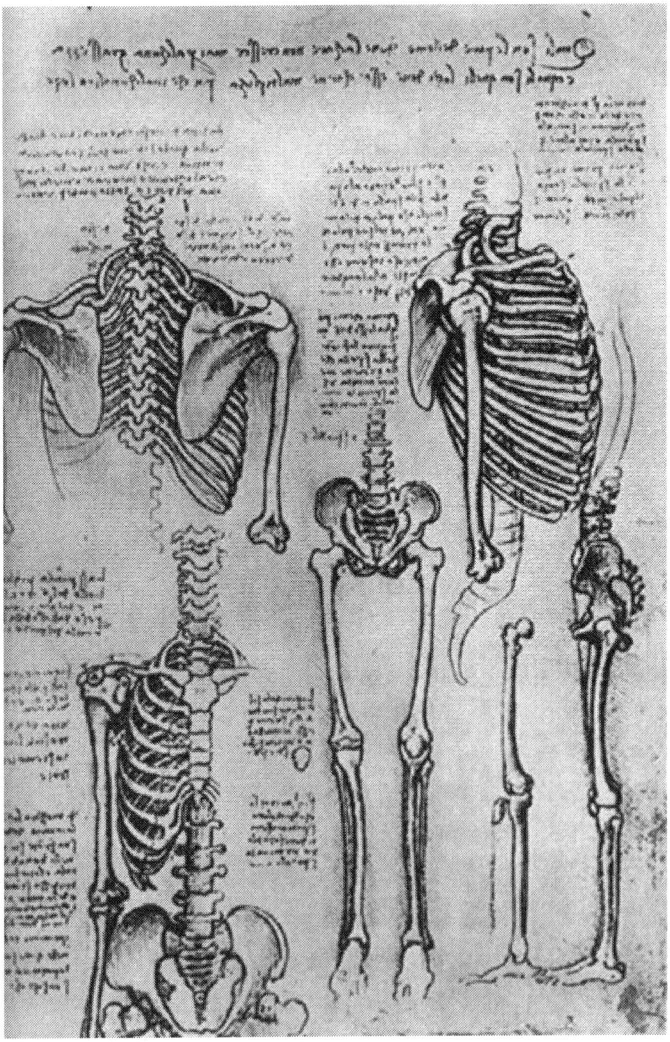

Figure 1C

His notes and drawings on this very subject were immense; they are still used as teaching aids for students in many different fields of study. They are considered by many to be the first detailed medical illustrations of the human body. Art students around the world use these drawings as reference material for their own work today. You can see his influence on how he perceived the world to be in our everyday life.

It was da Vinci that would go on to say that with each new human subject; we always need to begin with a firm foundation to build our masterpiece upon.

The human body's foundation begins with the skeleton; as we can see in da Vinci's illustration in Figure 1C, it's what he would describe as a grounding force to nature. One of the many different links to nature that we can use as a building block to form our body. This is where we can begin to find a design that has evolved over time, but began as one basic design.

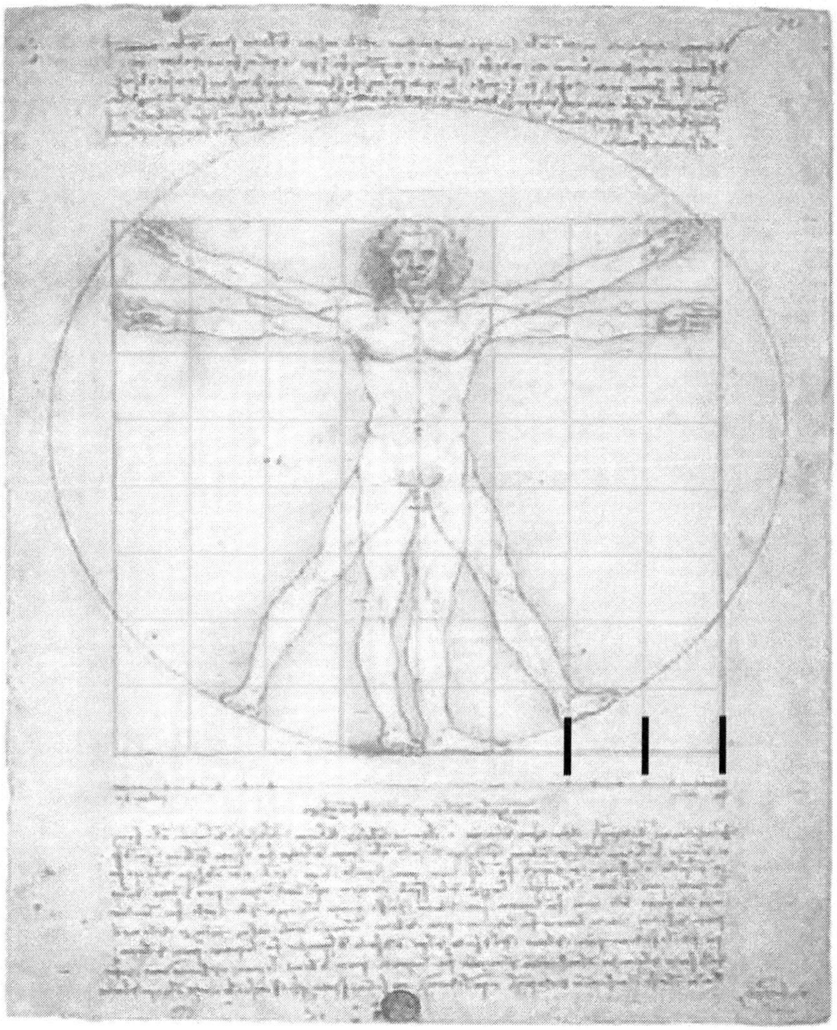

Figure 2C

To begin with, I think it's necessary to understand exactly what the dimensions of the Vitruvian Man were; described by Vitruvius and by da Vinci, not just the proportions in a scaled down version in a small drawing. To do that; let's first look at Figure 2C, and what those small squares really can tell us. In the description of the Vitruvian Man; among the notes that surround it, da Vinci says that 24 palms make a man, and we know also by this description that he says that it takes four fingers to make one palm; so if we were to measure four fingers we would find that it would measure approximately three inches. That would make the Vitruvian Man about 72 inches tall or approximately six feet tall; studies have shown that during the early Middle Ages the average height of an adult male was around 68 inches tall, so how does the drawing represent the basic proportions of a human body if the average is shorter than what da Vinci represents?

I believe da Vinci would use this measurement of a man's height because this is what Vitruvius described; and in order to discover what Vitruvius had described as the ideal proportions, da Vinci would first use the same measurements to better understand why Vitruvius would use them. It's exactly why at first I would use the same measurements that da Vinci described in his notes; I wanted to know what he knew. Vitruvius used these measurements because they are equally proportional to some of the same ratios he used in the buildings that he designed; but I don't want to use this for a common ratio to design a building, I want to find that one basic design of a human body.

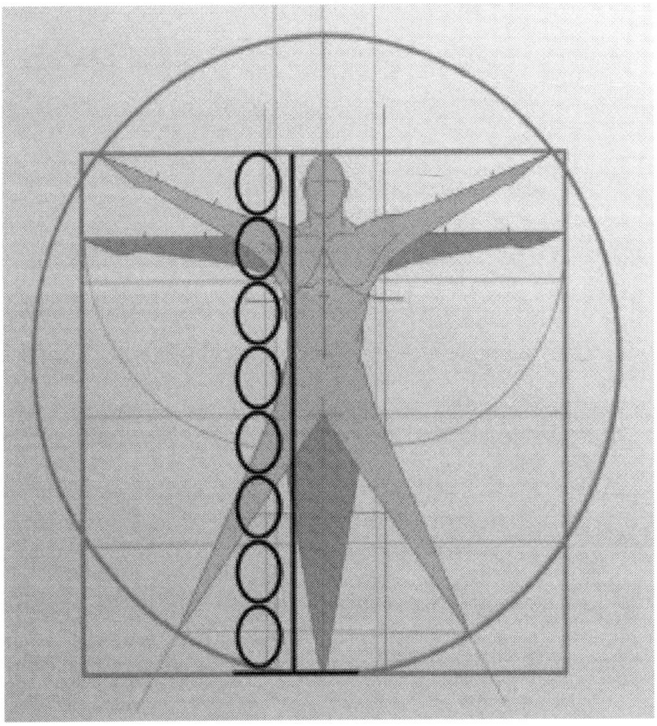

Figure 3C

If we look back at Figure 2C; we can see that this body is divided into 8 squares in length from the top of the head to the bottom of the feet; and one of these squares represents the length of the head, from the top of the head to the bottom of the chin. In Figure 3C, we can see how we could use the measurement of the head as a benchmark to find the height of that person; but there are several arguments that people aren't always 8 heads tall, and in fact they can range from anywhere between 7 heads tall to 8 heads tall. If that were true then there's really no way of finding this basic design. I don't think that's right; I think there's a basic benchmark for every human body, and I think that there are very few people that will fit perfectly into it. There are; and always will be, many different things that could lead our bodies away from that benchmark, because not one person will be perfect.

So how do we begin to find this benchmark that will work for anybody? Let's think of it like a math problem; if we have several different circles, all with different diameters, the one thing we know that can be used to find the areas of each one is to use the mathematical constant pi. If we look at Figure 4C, we see five completely different circles; and even though they are different sizes and different colors, the one thing they all have in common is that we can always find the area of each one if we use the constant pi. No matter what happens to their size, if it's a circle, then pi will always remain the same measurement, and it can be used as a benchmark to find the area.

Figure 4C

The constant, or benchmark, for the body is eight heads for any one body; and we can represent that as the body divided by eight parts to find the length of the head. Now we can create an equation that will help us find the length of the head.

$$b = \text{body height}$$

$$h = \text{head length}$$

$$\frac{b}{8} = h$$

We can use this equation to find the head length of the Vitruvian Man; it would be 72/8, which would equal a 9 inch head length. If we look again at Figure 2C; we can see that it's 3 palms in length, which would be 9 inches.

There have been many anthropological studies that have shown a correlation between the head length and the body height; but it's not exact for everyone within these studies. That could be because with each person there will be some form of divergence from this basic ratio; because there will always be some outside influence that will affect the ratio in some way or another. It could be something that might affect the head length that might also affect the overall ratio; or there might be something that could throw off the ratio of the rest of the body that would also affect the outcome of the whole body ratio. Something as insignificant as only 1/16 of inch difference in the measurement of the head length can make the whole system seem to not work. See Figure 5C.

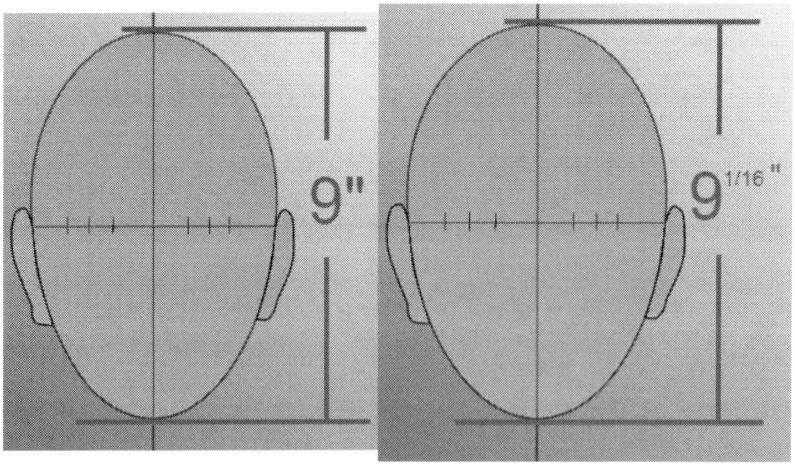

Figure 5C

This small difference in the head length will make a difference between one body being measured 72 inches and the other being measured 72.5 inches; that's at least a

½ inch for each 1/16 inch. That could mean a lot if the measurement of the head is off by just a little bit.

Even with all of the fancy measuring devices that can be used to more accurately measure the head; if the person being measured decided to open their mouth just by a little, moving their lower jaw down without it being noticed, could throw any study off by some margin. That's why this basic design has been disregarded as being anything thing that we can take seriously. It's also the reason why we haven't really noticed the difference in our everyday life; with the shape of the head it's harder to distinguish this difference at a glance. Look at Figure 6C.

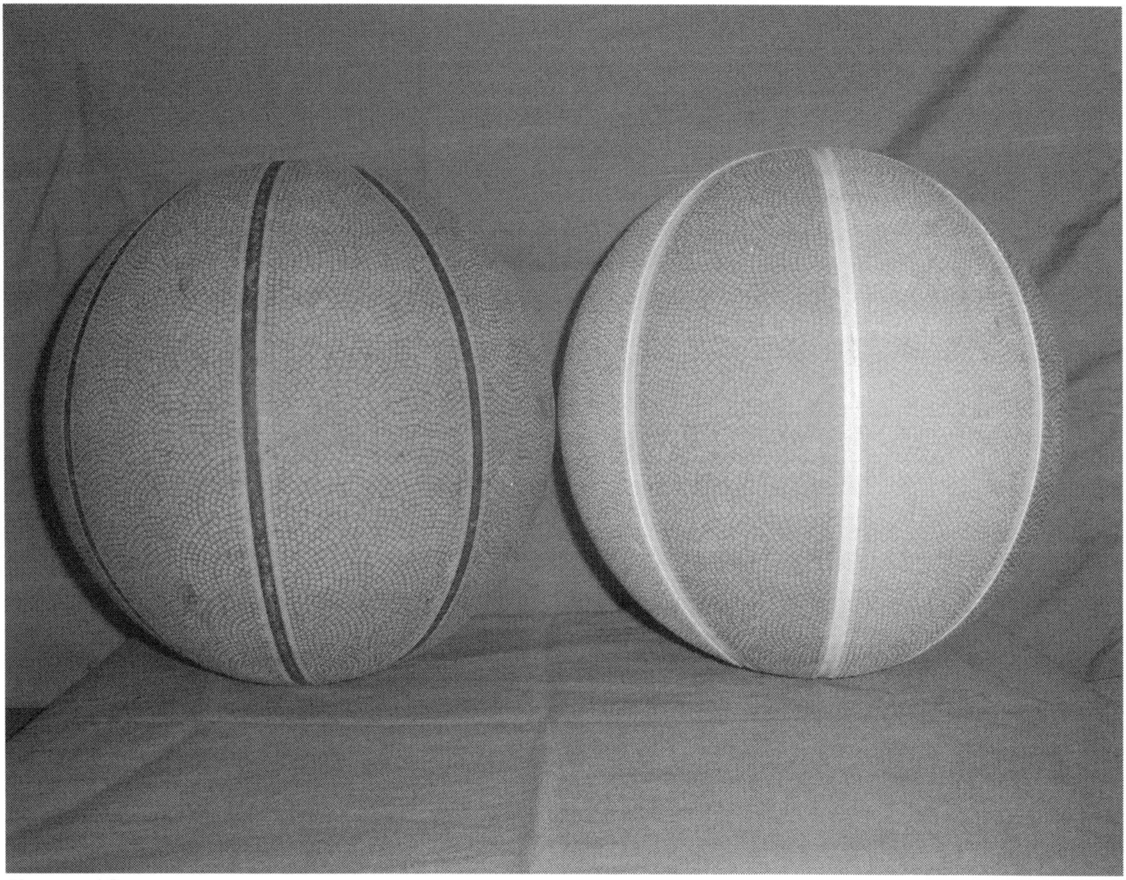

Figure 6C

These two basketballs are different sizes; one has been deflated by just a little bit, but even when they're setting side by side, it's hard to see the difference. The shape of a ball makes it harder to notice where the edge is; therefore making it harder to see which one is smaller, but if they were a different shape, like the cylinders in Figure 7C, then we can clearly see that difference.

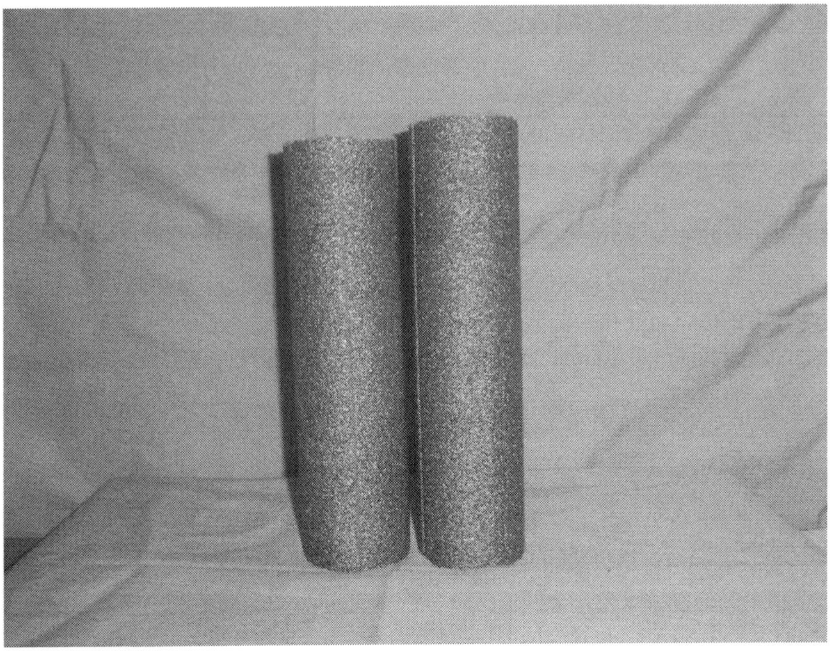

Figure 7C

These two are the same size as the basketballs; but as they're different shapes, we now see that one is taller than the other. This small difference; if they were actually two heads side by side; would be that one body would be about four inches taller than the other. The shape of the head is different than just a round ball; the lower jaw creates an edge that we can clearly distinguish, and therefore we should be able to use this as an edge that we can compare the differences of each head we see or measure.

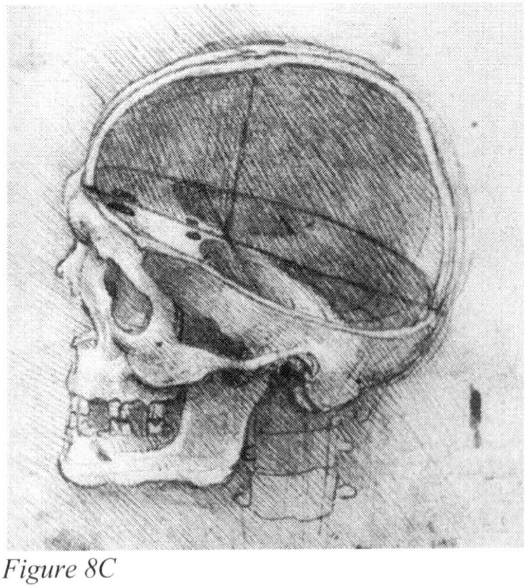

Figure 8C

You can clearly see the edge of the lower jaw in this da Vinci drawing of a skull; so why is it so hard to tell the difference if someone has a head slightly larger than someone else's head.

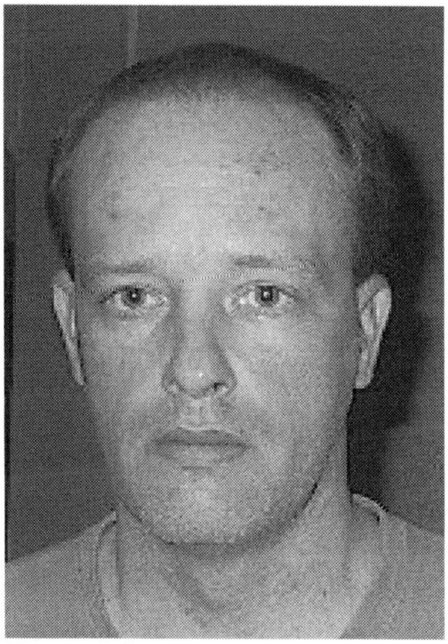

Figure 9C

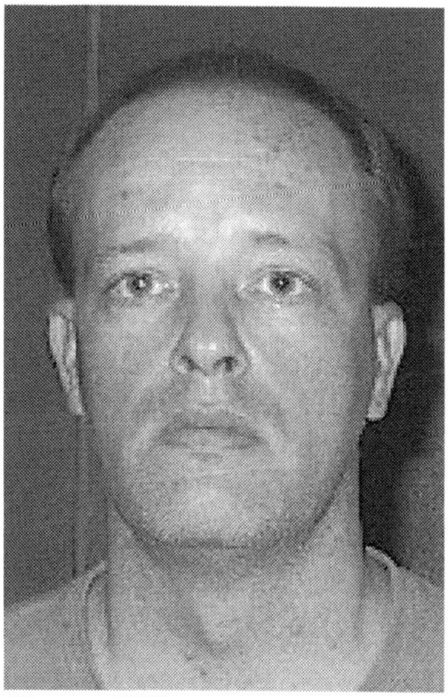

Figure 10C

The shape of the head is different than just a round ball; but the head is also shaped in a way that if you look at it at different angles, the head seems to change size. Look at Figures 9C and 10C, this is the same head; but at different angles the same head seems to have different measurements.

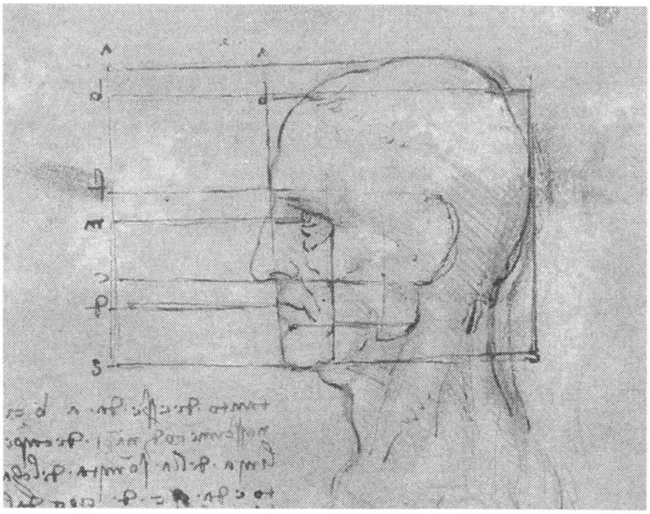

Figure 11C

This measurement has gone unseen throughout history because it's such a small value that it's been overlooked. The proportions of the rest of the whole body are so common; that such an insignificant value has been hidden within these proportions and we haven't really noticed it because it does seem so common. It's not something that looks out of place; because everything seems to go together so well, that unless it is measured accurately, our eyes will not notice the difference. In fact, most people hardly ever notice these little differences unless they're trained to spot these details. If you witness a crime and are asked to describe the suspect, most people will have a hard time trying to remember those small details that could pick the suspect out of the crowd; usually they will give only a general description of the person unless there is something really significant that stands out that makes the suspect different. This design can be seen well if we take a look at how to measure the head's proportions and how it relates to the body. We can see that da Vinci believed that there could be some way to find any key feature of the head; and that those same proportions could be used to draw anybody's head, no matter who they might be. In Figure 11C, we can see by his sketch how he would make notes about these proportions; but he would have also seen that in real life these proportions may not work for everybody, so he would describe a basic design as a starting point to begin his drawings, and then he could make any necessary adjustments needed to each individual.

The most basic design of the human is what most artists will always begin with; and it's defined as an oval shape with two eyes, one mouth, one nose, two ears, and most of the time, with hair on top. This is a definitive description of the human head; the basic design. Look at Figure 12C.

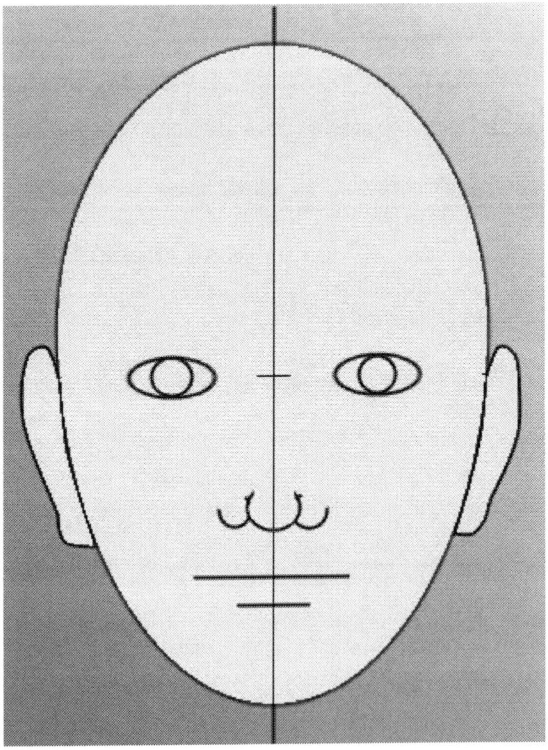

Figure 12C

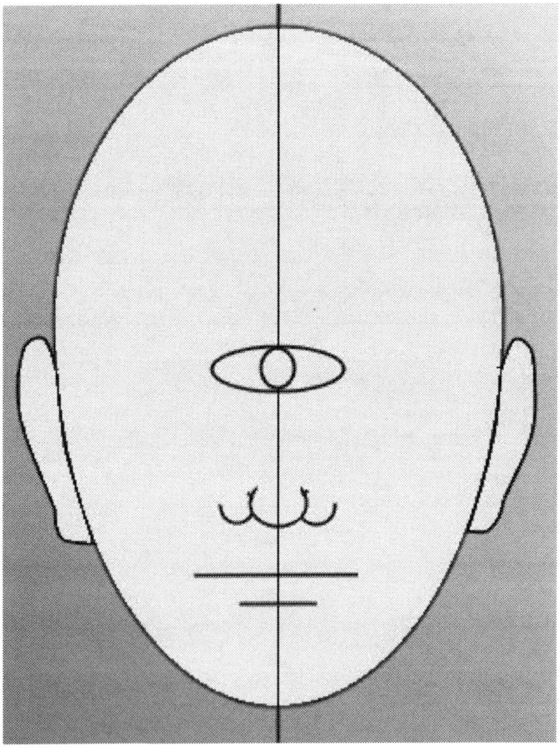

Figure 13C

Even if there is one thing off the list of what we consider to be a human head; like in Figure 13C, we would take notice right away. The person in Figure 13C would be considered a mutation to what we would think of as normal. It wouldn't be considered a natural occurrence. You may not think about it; but we all know this basic design, and we can tell if there is something off what we consider to be our natural proportions. The way our body grows doesn't affect this proportion either; even if one person is taller than the next, they both still have that same proportion.

Even though the square on the left in Figure 14C is larger than the one on the right; they still both have the same proportions, they each have four smaller squares contained within them. The same thing would occur with two different people of different heights. This would be the basic design that da Vinci would have tried to relate to each individual, except that each person might have a slight difference in one ratio because of some outside force that has pushed them away from that basic ratio.

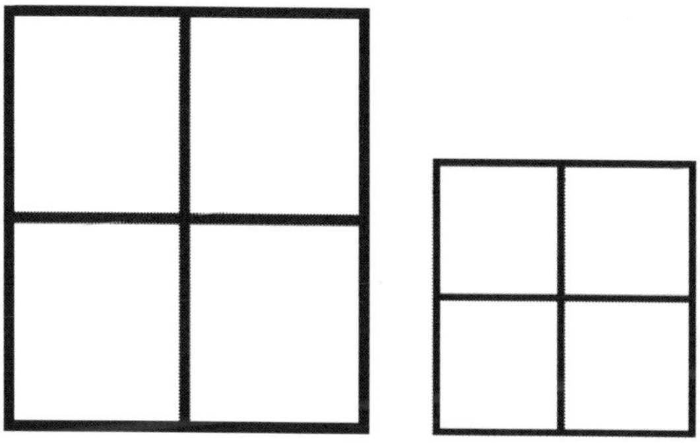

Figure 14C

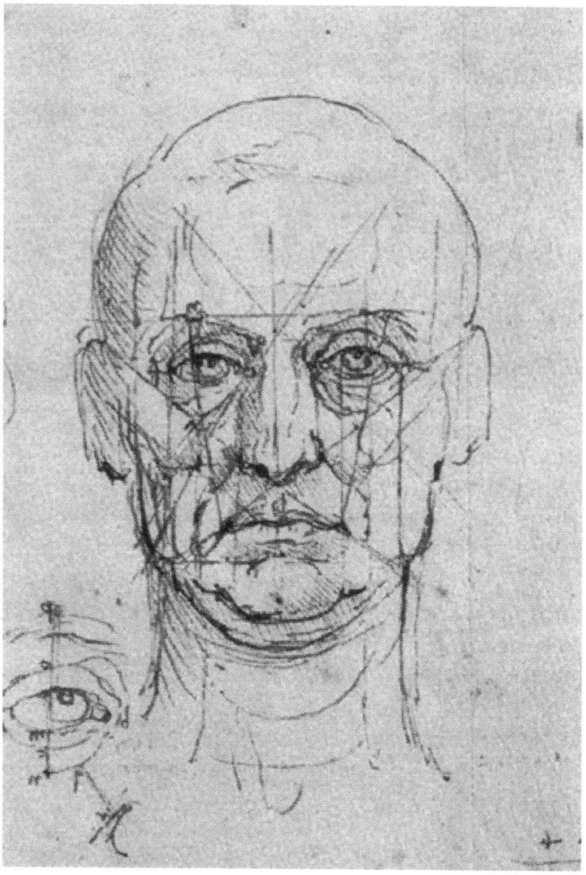

Figure 15C

In Figure 15C, da Vinci's study of the proportions of the head seems to show how the head has a form of symmetry to it as compared to the design of the eye; but the head doesn't start out with this same symmetry.

When we are born, as mentioned before, our body is at a 1 to 4 ratio with the skull that's not completely formed. The facial features, such as the brow, nose, and the jawbone; haven't still fully developed either. After birth and along with the skull, these features will rapidly begin to develop its own individualized form. The facial features of the skull seem to develop quicker at this time than the circumference of the skull. The face at this time looks more flat and the features are less defined.

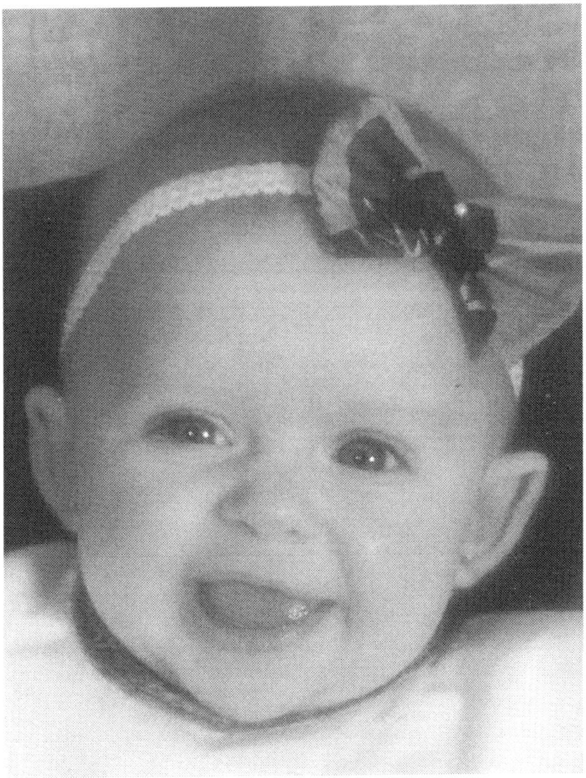

Figure 16C

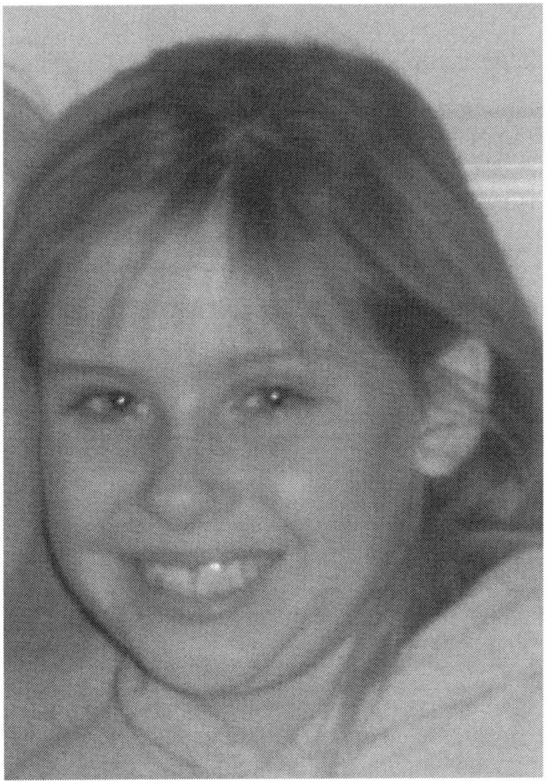

Figure 17C

The picture in Figure 16C is of a baby at about 3 to 6 months old, and as we can see; the facial features have not fully developed yet. The picture of the girl in Figure 17C is the same girl as in Figure 17C; except now she is 9 years old. If we compare the two photos, we can see the differences in the shape of the head.

In Figure 18C; her forehead is narrower at the top. "The bones of the roof the skull are initially separated by regions of dense connective tissue called "fontanels". [8] This makes it easier for the plates to move around; making it easier for birth. The plates will then move closer to each other to form a more solid form, and then these fontanels will become sutures. Soon after birth; the head seems to be more rounded at the top.

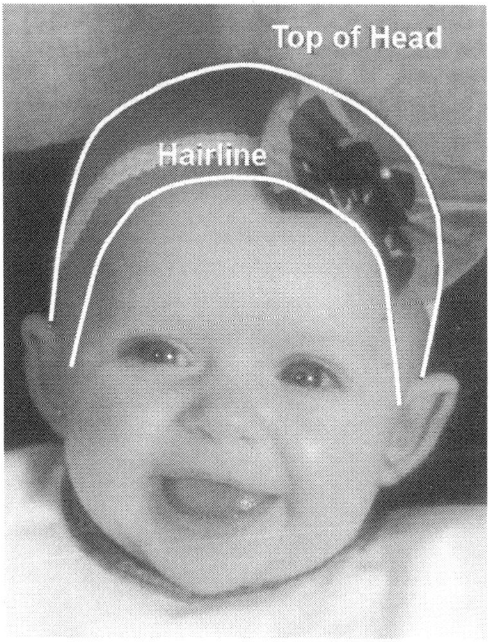

Figure 18C

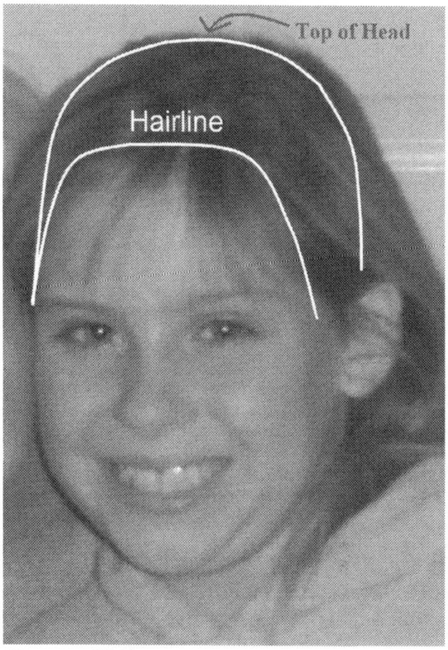

Figure 19C

As we grow the head will form a more block like form, as seen in Figure 19C. The hairline will also push outwards as we grow; you can see the difference between the two Figures, this will make the head into a more rounded form, like the one in Figure 19C.

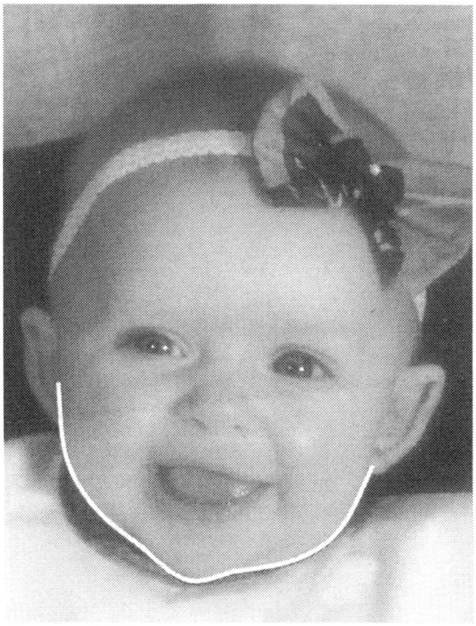

Figure 20C

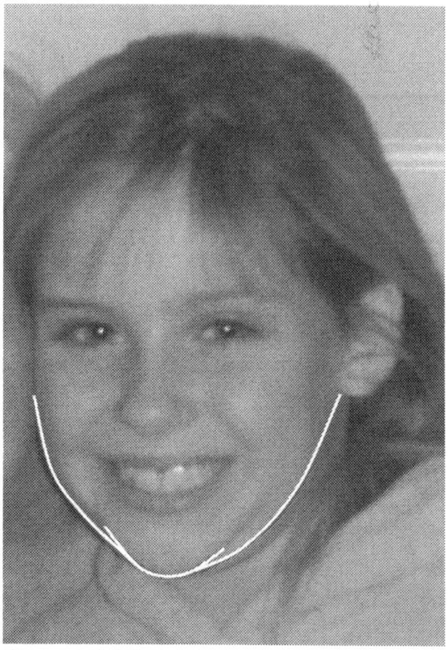

Figure 21C

The jaw line is another significant key feature that changes over time. One study shows that mandible may move forward as much as 10mm within the first 3 years after birth. As you can see; the overall shape changes also. It begins to form a more pointed shape in a flat photograph. When we look at these flat photographs, we need to remember that we are looking at a three dimensional shape that has been flatten by the camera and no matter how good the camera is, there will always be some distortion.

Now we need to look at how the brow seems to push outwards. The all important eyebrows call this region home. The brow is also connected to the top of the nasal bridge between the eyes. This region seems to also push outwards as we grow.

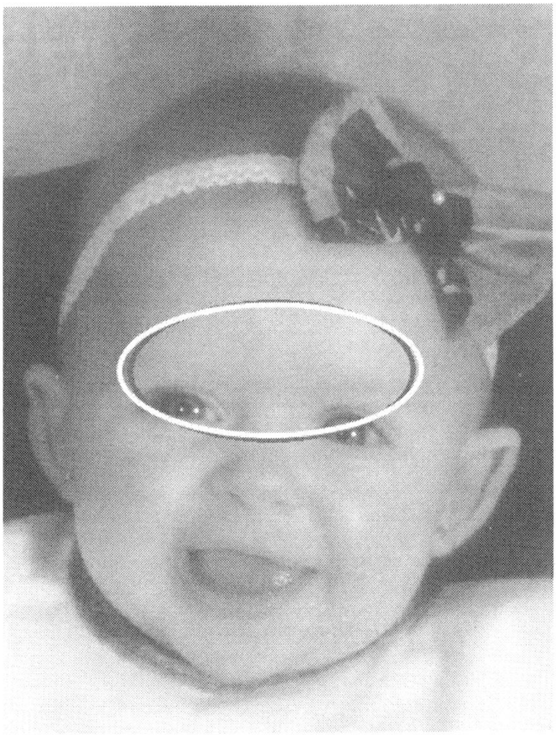

Figure 22C

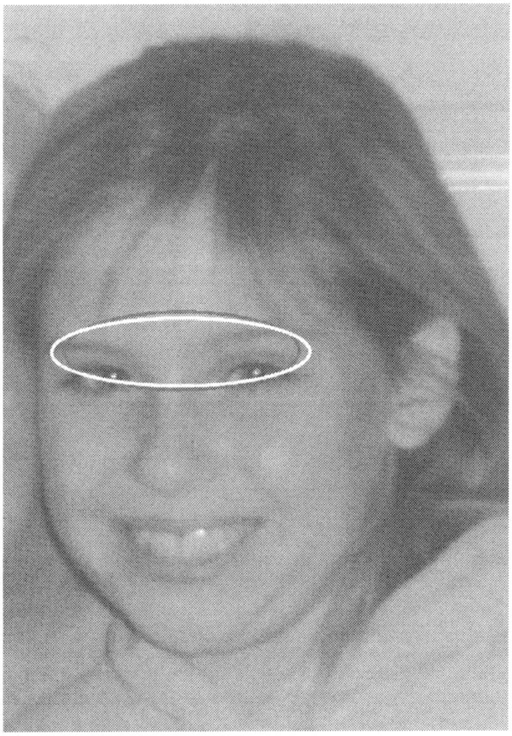

Figure 23C

We can also see how the nasal bridge pushes outward. The face doesn't seem as flat within this region as the facial features become more defined. See Figure 23C, the nose begins to have a more block like form. The eyes begin to look pushed back into the face, but instead the brow is beginning to push out. You can see it growing out in Figure 24C.

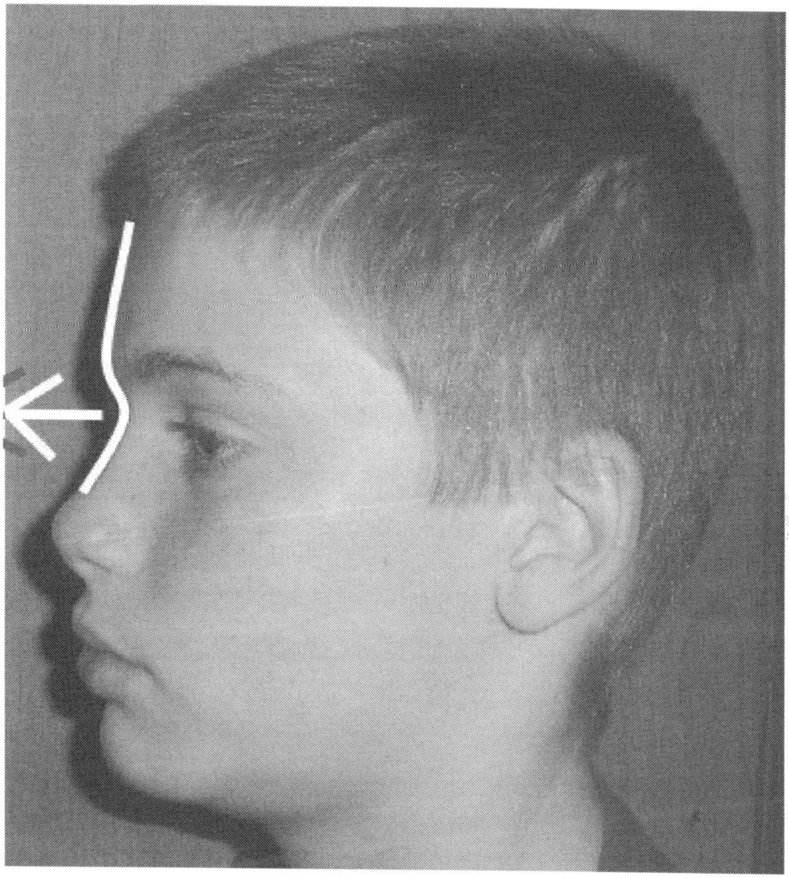

Figure 24C

I believe we can recognize this feature without thinking about it, and we associate it with growing older. This is a feature that when a person looks at these two features, in a photograph or in person, we know that a person, like in Figure 22C, is a small child and that a person, like in Figure 23C, is an older child. I don't think that a lot of people recognize this difference because we see it every day and therefore it just becomes second nature to associate it as such. These are small differences we associate with growing older; but without the wrinkles it seems to go unnoticed, we know there's a difference, but we seem to just accept that since the body as a whole is growing, we don't have to notice these smaller differences.

There's one more key feature to look at: the eyes. The old saying, "The eyes are the windows to the souls." Well this may or may not be correct, but they could be the windows to the proportions of the face, or at least a way to measure those features. So, how do we use the eyes as a way to measure and why do we use the eye as a standard to measure with?

Let's answer the question of why we'll use the eyes as a standard measure. We'll need to begin by describing how the eye grows. As mentioned before, "Height and weight show rapid growth in infancy and puberty and show 'S-type' growth patterns, whereas brain, head circumference, and visual organs are of the neural type and grow up to 80% of the adult size by age 4." [9] The brain, head circumference, and the visual organs are of the neural type, and therefore should grow at the same rate. The eye should grow at the same rate as the skull, because if the skull grew at a different rate, then the eyeball would not fit in the skull at different times of growth. "By and large the growth of the eye follows the growth pattern of the brain." [13] It will remain in the eye socket of the skull with the same fit throughout your life; that is if nothing is wrong.

If it grows at the same rate, then why do the eyes look larger when we're infants? There is a small, but important feature of the eye that's largely overlooked when we look at other people. Have you ever noticed the corners of the eyes and how they're shaped? Have you really looked how the eyelids come together? Let's look at a closer view of the eyes of Figure 16C and Figure 17C.

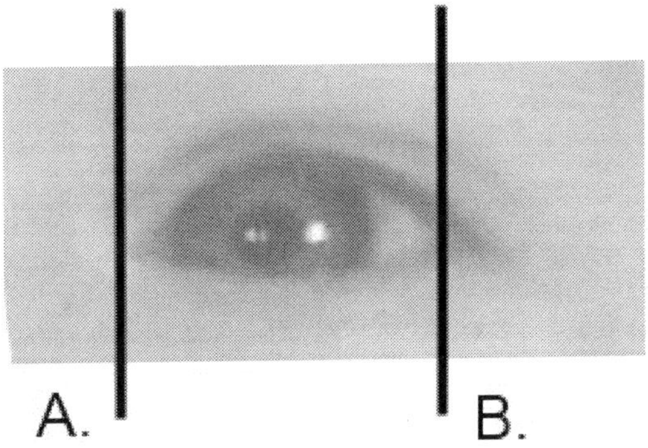

Figure 25C

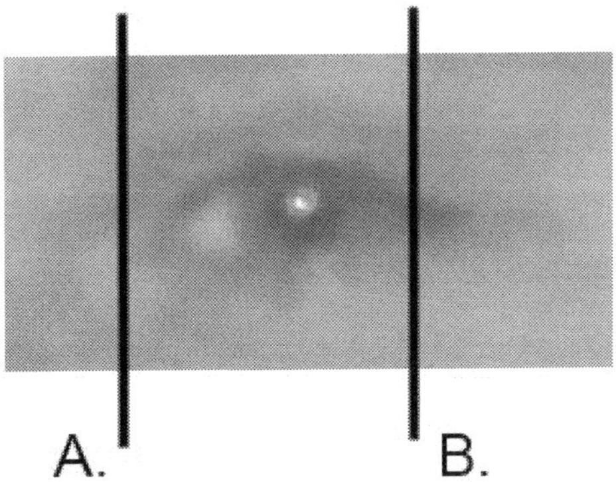

Figure 26C

Figure 25C is a closer version of Figure 16C and Figure 26C is a closer version of Figure 17C. The medial commissure on both Figures 25C and 26C are represented by the letter A.; this is where the eyelids meet together closer to the nose. The letter B. is the lateral commissure; it's closer to the temple. As we grow older, it seems the medial commissure gets a little longer. Why is that? As the skull, brow, and nose begin to develop; the eye grows at the same rate, but the skin around the eye seems to stretch, therefore exposing the eye slightly more as we grow. We can see a bigger difference in the shape of the medial commissure as the skin stretches. It's worthwhile to see these subtle differences; it's how we process these differences that tell us if the eye is a young eye or an older eye. If we look at it from a different angle, we can see how the medial commissure stretches along the ridge of the nose. The ridge of the nose in Figure 27C is at an adult size, but you can see how far the skin will have to stretch in order to get to its destination. See Figure 27C.

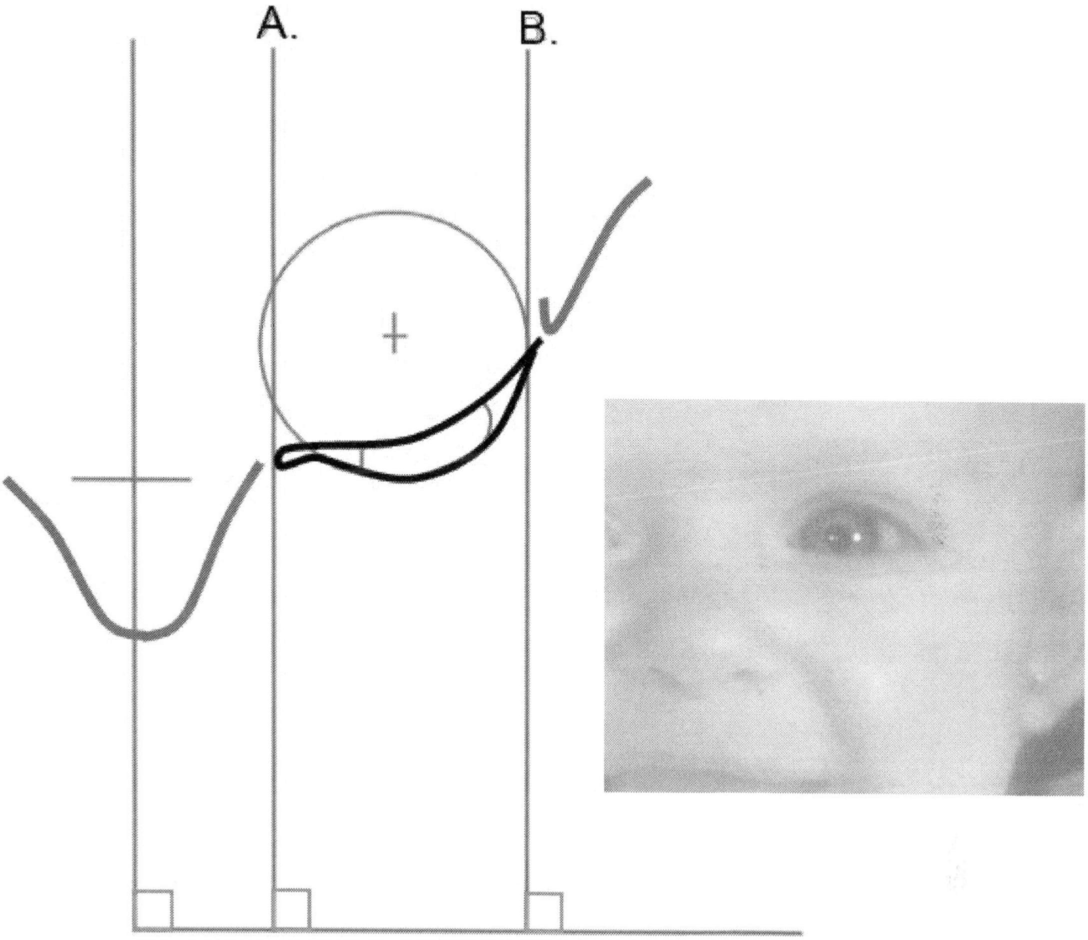

Figure 27C

In Figure 27C, it's a representation of the eye of the infant in Figure 16C. The letter A. represents the medial commissure and B. represents the lateral commissure. Notice where A. is in comparison with the middle of the nose, now look at the same thing in Figure 28C. The representation of the eye in Figure 28C is the same as the eye in Figure 17C. As you can tell; after looking at the different drawings, there is only a slight movement of the commissure, but it's enough to make a difference when trying to represent a younger eye versus an older eye. It's also small enough to go unnoticed, unless you look closely.

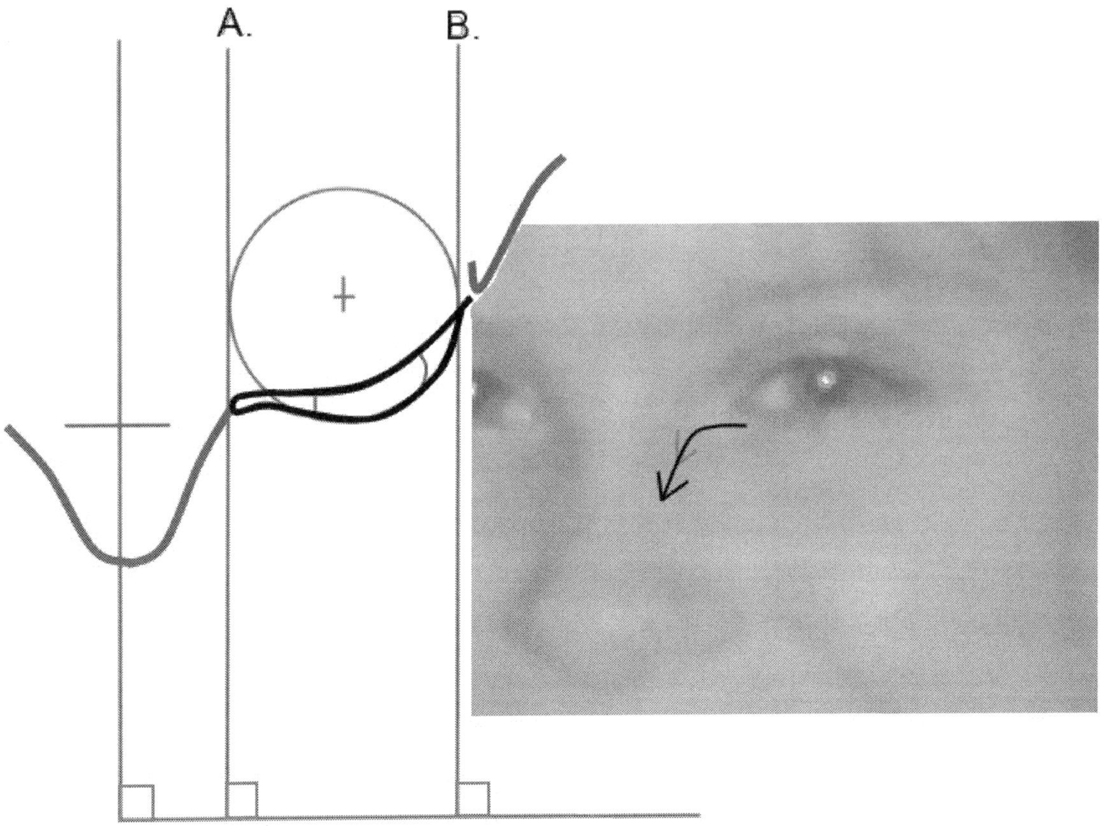

Figure 28C

See how the medial commissure stretches along the inside of the ridge of the nose? As the ridge of the nose grows, the skin will form along with the nose, stretching the eyelids, therefore exposing the eye a little more as we grow older. The rate of growth of the eyeball stays at this proportion, because in order for it to fit in the eye socket it would have to stay at this same proportion.

Another reason why it seems as though the eyes tend to look larger soon after birth is how the iris is proportioned as compared to the rest of the eye.

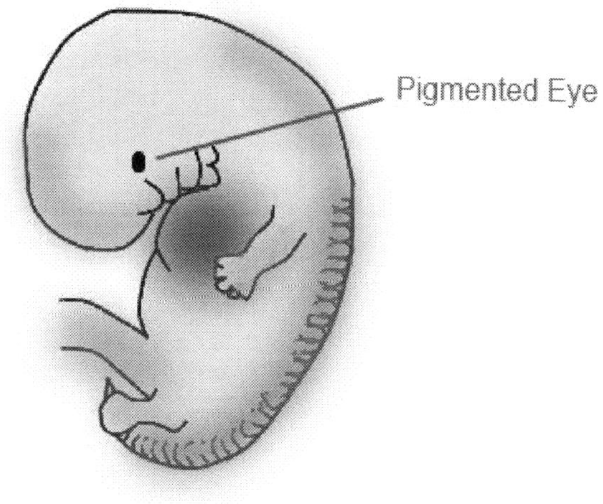

Figure 29C

At about six weeks of the development of the human embryo, we can start to see the pigmented eye; which would lead us to believe that the iris has began development before the sclera, or maybe we can see this development before we can see the development before the sclera. The development of the eye stock behind this pigmented eye will give us a clue to why the iris seems to be larger than the rest of the eye.

As the eye grows within the eye socket of the skull; the sclera will grow at the same

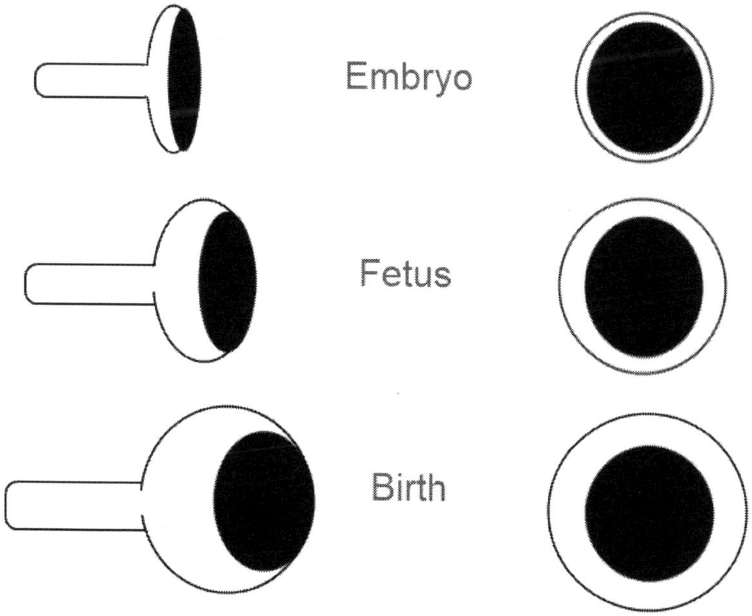

Figure 30C

The measurement of the eye has proven to be the undoing of how we perceive that this whole body proportion seems to be wrong with each individual person; because if you do measure the eye, it doesn't seem to conform to these proportions. "When we remove the eye from the orbit, we can see that the eye is a slightly asymmetrical sphere with an approximate saggital diameter or length of 24 to 25 mm and a transverse diameter of 24 mm." [14] When we measure the eye while in the eye socket surrounded by the eyelids; measured from the inner corner of the eye to the outer corner of the eye, it has a proportion of eight eye lengths to one head length.

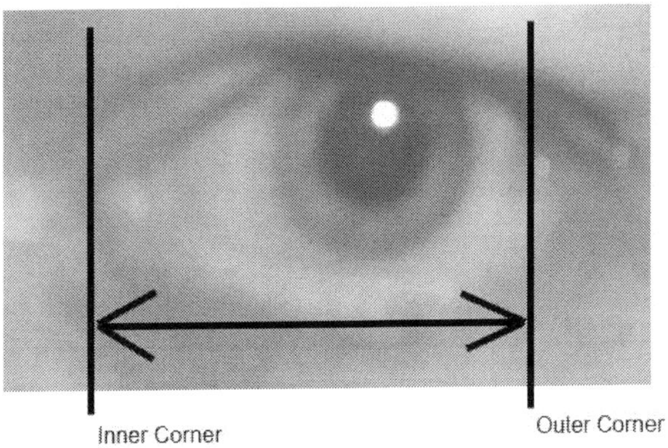

Figure 31C

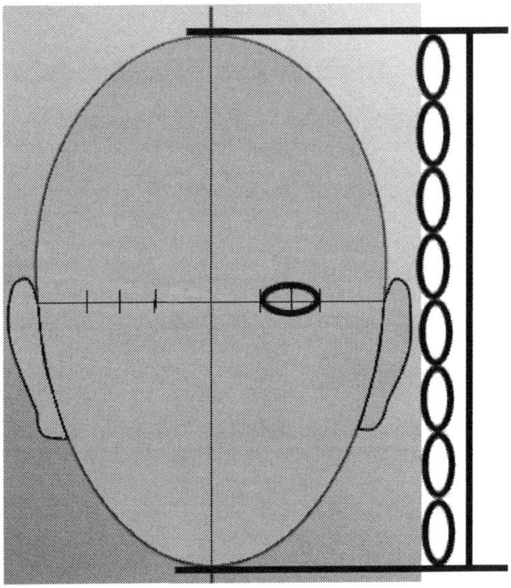

Figure 32C

The eye within the eye socket isn't always easy to measure; it will take on a completely different shape than just a rounded ball to measure. The eye has a shape that will measure differently if you measure it at different angles. This measurement is a combination of a circular outline and a small a curve on the end. From the top view, we can see that it looks more like the shaped of a cup holding the eyeball in its place. This shape makes it more difficult to get the same results every time; unless you measure it at the same angle every time you measure. Let's take a look at Figures 33C and 34C to get a better idea of how this works.

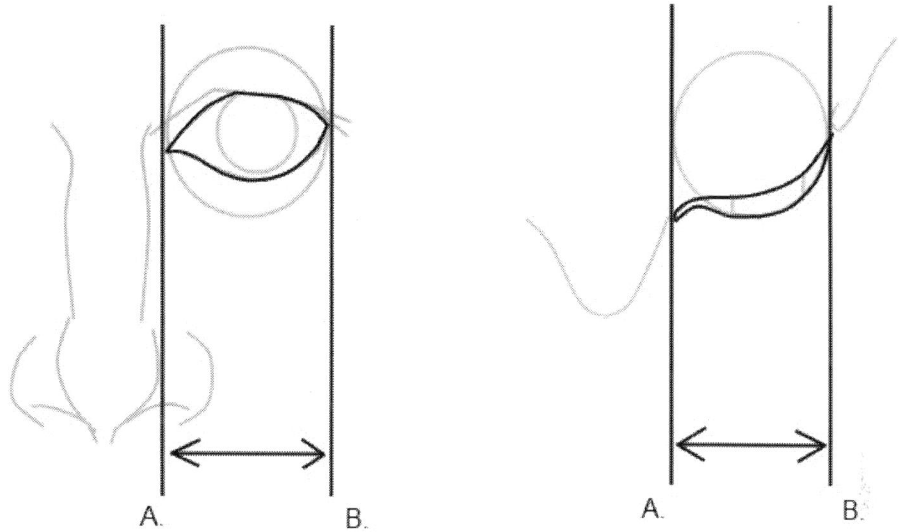

Figure 33C

If you measure the eye; looking directly at you, this measurement from point A. to point B. will be the median measurement. If you look at this odd shape from the top, as in Figure 33C, you can see how it pushes outward towards the ridge of the nose. This measurement; as you measure it from another angle will grow at first, and then it will shrink. Take a look at Figure 34C; and you can see that the measurement from point A. to point B. has increased in size. It's because of its odd shape; after this point it will begin to decrease in size. It will decrease as much as over half the size measured in Figure 33C.

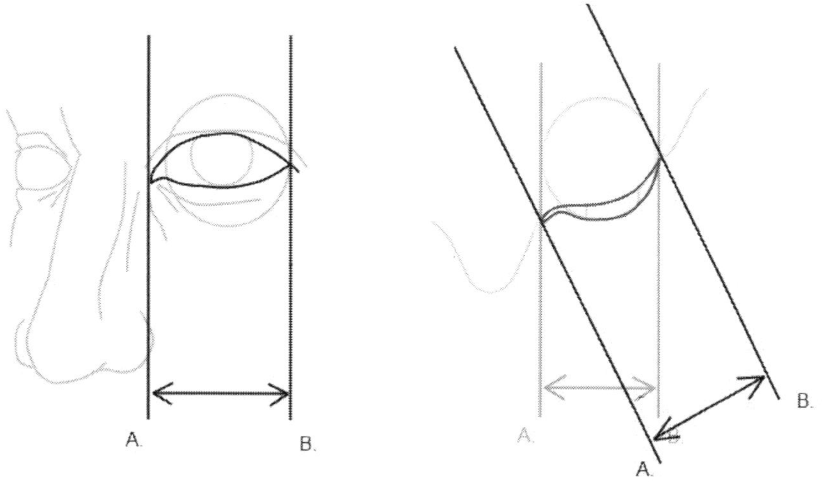

Figure 34C

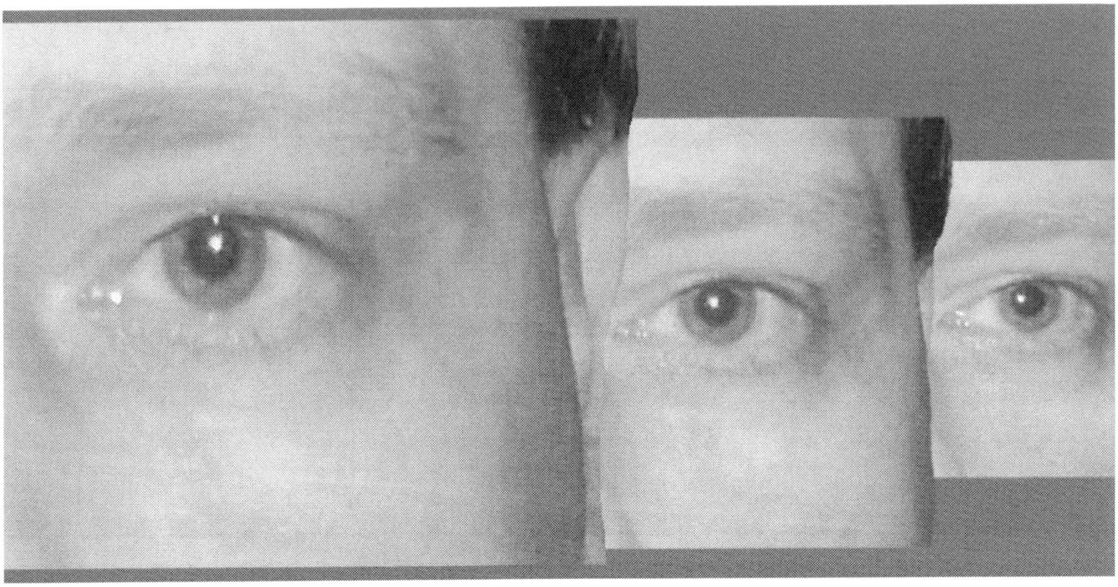

Figure 35C

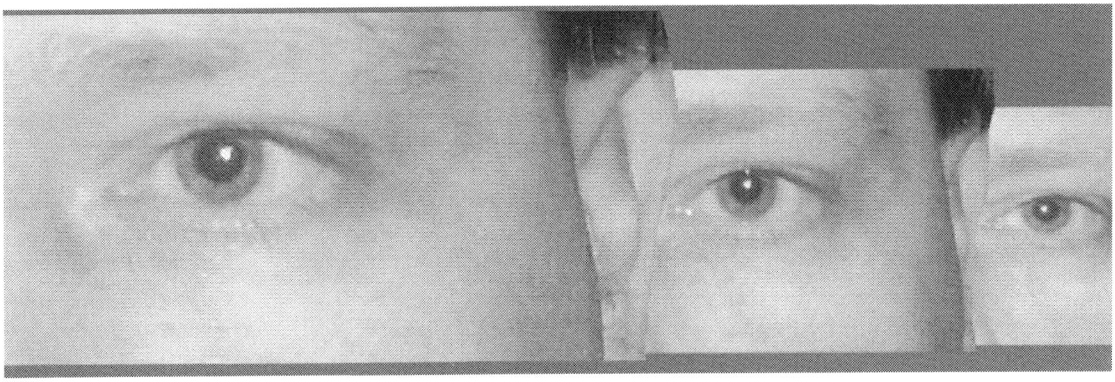

Figure 36C

In Figures 35C and 36C, you can see how it changes with different angles. The difference is at the outer corner; look at it and see how it changes.

We've seen how the eye changes measurement at different angles; and we know that the head measurement can be affected by the angle in which it is measured, so how can we find that median measurement for the head?

First we need to establish the best angle for the head to be measured by; and then use this measurement to find that individual's median measurement. The head needs to be looking directly ahead, and the head shouldn't be turned or tilted. If we examine the photo in Figure 37C; we see that the head is the best position to measure this median. Point P. is at the spot where the ear is attached to the head; this line should be even with the outer corner of the eye. Point Q. is at the bottom side of the ear, and that line should be even with the bottom of the nose.

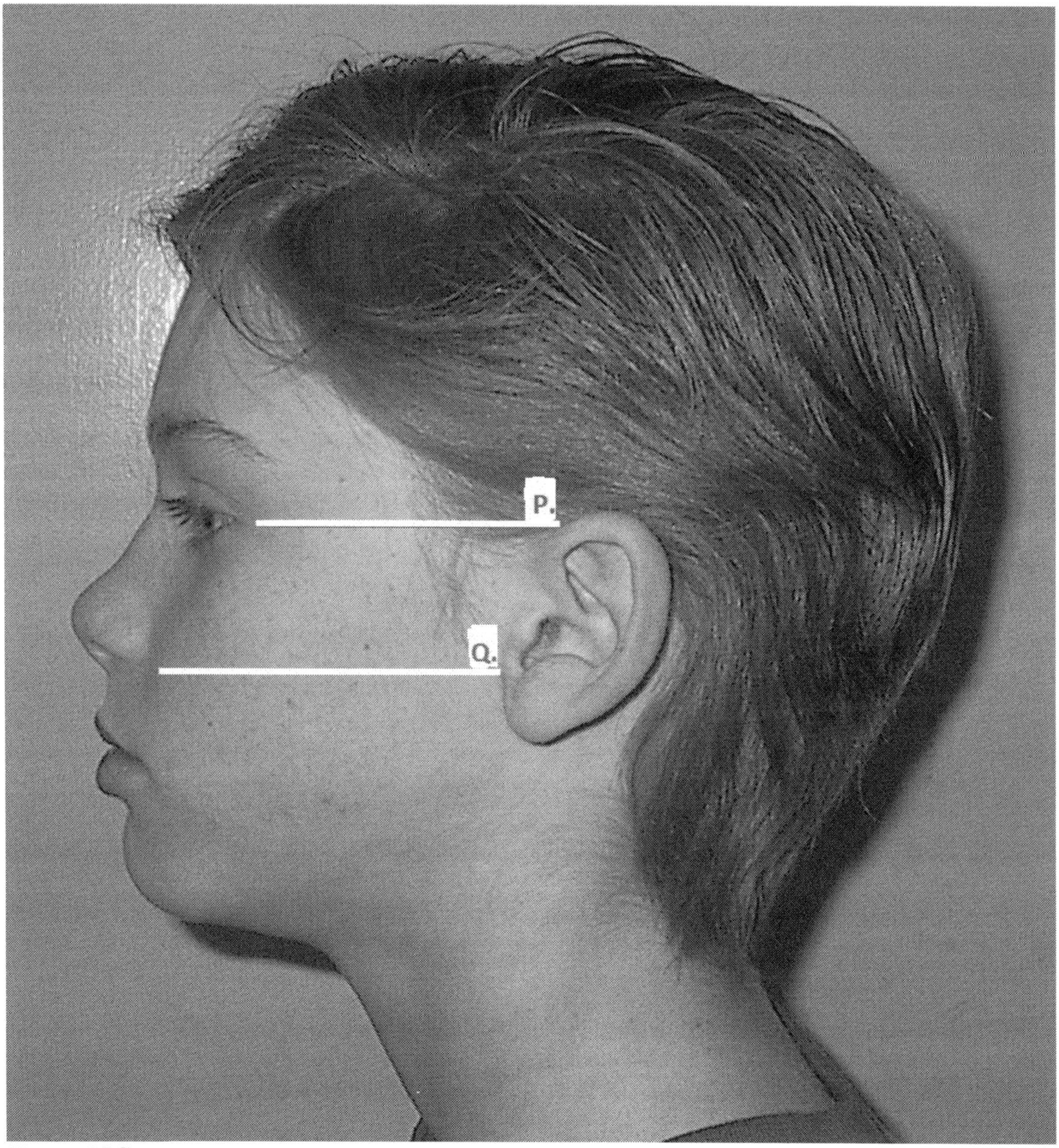

Figure 37C

If we use these established guidelines; then we can measure the basic form of the body and its proportions, and we can find how far away that body has veered away from that measurement.

The Original Design

I think its possible da Vinci may have been searching for this one basic design of a human body; and I also believe he was looking for the one design that we began with. This design would be the form that we all evolved from; the one form that we all deviate from, no matter where we come from. He wouldn't just be looking for the general form and its ratios; I think he was searching for what the very first human would have looked like.

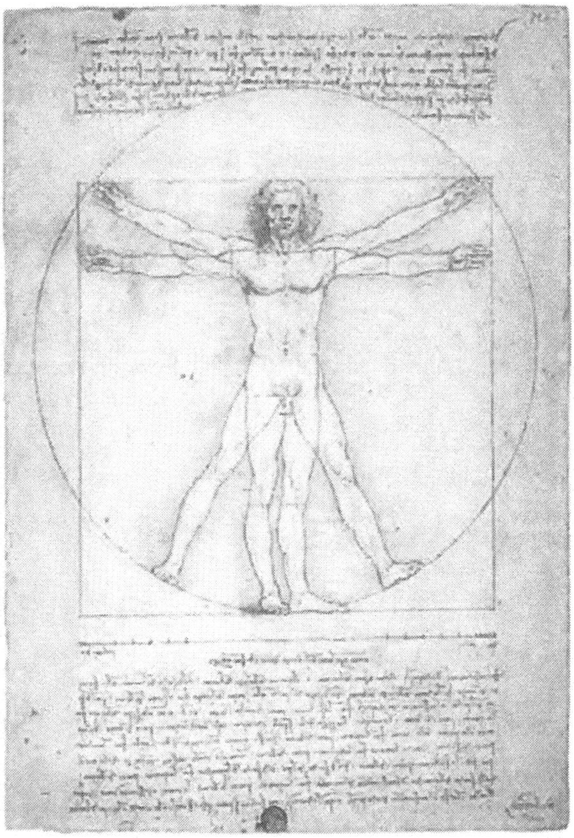

Figure 1D

He didn't just stop here with the drawing of the Vitruvian Man; this was only the beginning for him, you can see his journey in all the extensive notes and all the different studies he made about the human body.

When we first began to explore the Vitruvian Man; we read what da Vinci said that Vitruvius had written in his books about architecture, "Vitruvius, the architect, says in his work on architecture that the measurements of the human body are distributed by Nature as follows: that is that 4 fingers make 1 palm and 4 palms make 1 foot, 6 palms make 1 cubit; 4 cubits make a man's height. And 4 cubits make one pace and 24 palms make a man; and these measures he used in his building."[7] He mentions three words; architect, architecture, and building, when he describes what Vitruvius wrote about an ideal proportioned man. He also goes on to mention that these measurements are distributed by Nature. At this time in history there were no well established universal units of measurement; there wasn't some standard unit that was being used by everyone. There were no tape measures or even standard rulers to measure with; and to have a measurement not equal a whole unit, that would be even harder to keep those measurements the same every time.

In those architecture books written by Vitruvius; he describes every little detail that an architect might encounter. The idea of symmetry and proportions were valued enough for the building of temples; that he would use a whole chapter about it. He would write that symmetry was so important; that an architect must pay it careful observation, and it's with proportions that we have symmetry. He would go on to say, "Without symmetry and proportion there can be no principles in the design of any temple; that is, if there is no precise relation between its members, as in the case of those of a well shaped man."[4] He believed that there could be no other design made by nature that could provide a better example of proportions than the human body. After he went on about what he thought those proportions should be; the same proportions da Vinci would later use, he would then talk about how a rule from the ancients was correct. He wrote, "Therefore, since nature has designed the human body so that its members are duly proportioned to the frame as a whole, it appears that the ancients had good reason for their rule, that in perfect buildings the different members must be in exact symmetrical relations to the whole general scheme. Hence, while transmitting to us the proper arrangements for buildings of all kinds, they were particularly careful to do so in the case of temples of the gods, buildings in which merits and faults usually last forever."[4] He was telling us that the buildings the ancients built for their gods paid particularly close attention to staying within the same proportions as a human body; because the buildings were so important to the common people. There would be vast crowds walking through them every day; important ceremonies would be held there, and so this building would be scrutinized so much, that the architect needed to pay special attention to these proportions.

Vitruvius would then surmise that it was from the members of that body that would be used by the ancients as their units of measure; the fingers, palms, foot, and cubit. He said that the ancients were fixed upon this perfect number of ten; because the members of the body were proportioned according to this perfect number. He wrote, "For it is from the number of the fingers of the hand that the palm is found, and the foot from the palm. Again, while ten is naturally perfect, as being made up by the fingers of the two palms, Plato also held that this number was perfect because ten is composed of the individual units, called by the Greeks μονάδες. But as soon as eleven or twelve is reached, the numbers, being excessive, cannot be perfect until they come to ten for the second time; for the component parts of that number are the individual units."[4] This number of ten was the ancients standard of measuring in their time; but then the mathematicians would try to prove this number not to be perfect, and would say that the number six was the more perfect number.

Vitruvius would then write, "The mathematicians, however, maintaining a different view, have said that the perfect number is six,"[4] After showing us how the ancient Greeks would use this number; he then go on to describe units of measure as they are compared to the human body. He wrote, "And further, as the foot is one sixth of a man's height, the height of the body as expressed in number of feet being limited to six, they held that this was the perfect number, and observed that the cubit consisted of six palms or of twenty-four fingers."[4] This was a description of how to find the perfect measurement for a foot. You need to find a person that is exactly six feet tall; and since the foot should be one sixth of the perfect proportions of a body, then if you measure that person's foot, it will be the correct measurement of one unit of measure, the foot.

He says in the book that his countrymen (the Romans); would at first use the ancient rule of ten, but then they would find that the number six looked even better as a more perfect number. "But later, observing that six and ten were both of them perfect numbers, they combined the two, and thus made the most perfect number, sixteen. They found their authority for this in the foot. For if we take two palms from the cubit, there remains the foot of four palms; but the palm contains four fingers. Hence the foot contains sixteen fingers,"[4] He is describing to the architect; not only the numbers they use, but how those numbers come about. He was trying to explain the method of why these units are so important, and how to find them.

"Therefore, if it is agreed that number was found out from the human fingers, and that there is a symmetrical correspondence between the members separately and the entire form of the body, in accordance with a certain part selected as standard, we can have nothing but respect for those who, in constructing temples of the immortal gods, have so arranged the members of the works that both the separate parts and the whole design may harmonize in their proportions and symmetry."[4]

He was explaining why it so important to use these proportions; and this is why da Vinci would begin by stressing this key of units that Vitruvius had written about in those architecture books. Those measurements are what da Vinci would use in measuring the human body; but we can also see that he would use what was called a braccio, an Italian measurement of the forearm. He would use this measurement for most of his drawings, especially for his mechanical and architecture drawings. This measurement is also the Italian approximation for the cubit; if we take into account what Vitruvius described, then we can see that it measures about 18 inches. You can in some of his drawings where he would draw a small arm; bent as to measure only the forearm.

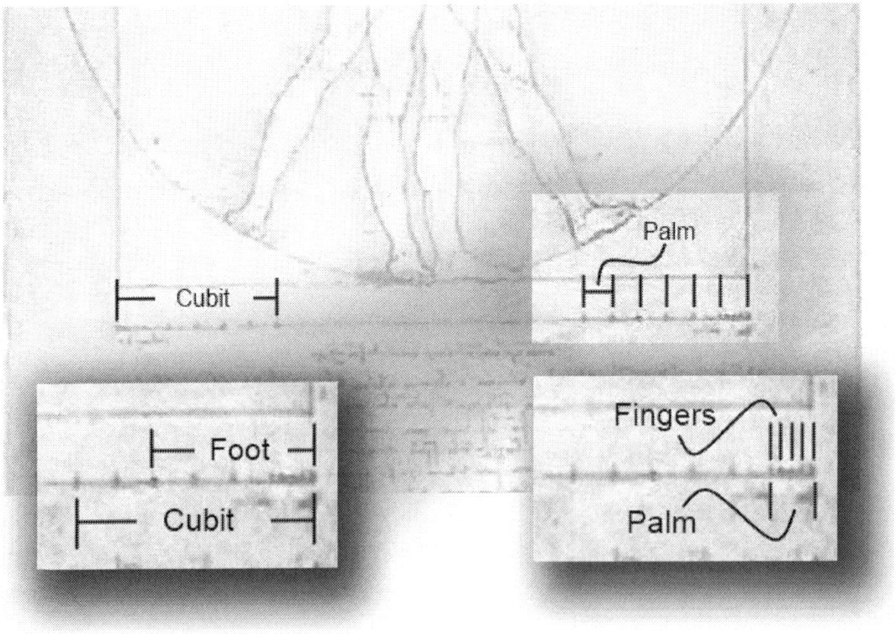

Figure 2D

We can take another look at this key on the Vitruvian Man, and see how the unit of the foot would be compared to the unit of cubits. In Figure 2D, we can see that the foot is about four palms, or 12 inches. The Vitruvian Man was built by the foot; a six foot man to be more precise, and it was from constructing a diagram of a man that is six feet tall, that we should find any proportioned measurement for all those units of measurements described by Vitruvius. The description of what has been called the ideal man; is really just a key to use for finding out what each unit of measurement; described by Vitruvius, should be measured.

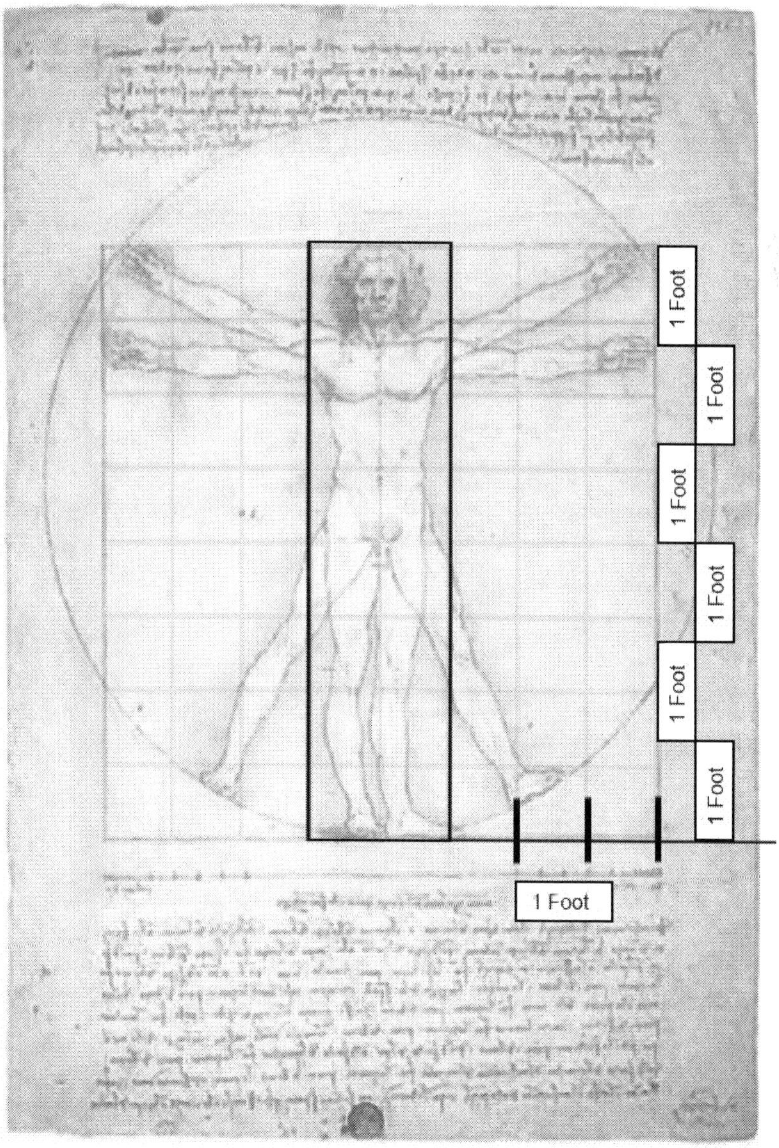

Figure 3D

In Figure 3D, we can see how the measurement of what was described by Vitruvius as one foot; would be compared to the drawing made by da Vinci.

This would give them a more precise way to find the length of anything; besides just relying on what a body part that measures differently with each individual. Now when they want to know how long a pace might be; they would measure it from a six foot tall man; but how did they know which person had reached six feet tall? Did Vitruvius use a model to establish this, because he had no idea how to first distinguish who was six feet tall. He first would have had to decide how tall six feet would be.

I think this is what would drive da Vinci to try to find that first original model of what a human body might measure. From this model he could then say for sure that one man is six feet, or that another might be five feet tall. This would establish exactly what all the other measurements would be compared to; to find out what this model might be, we need to describe what that person could have look like.

To start with, we need to find the first model of the body; and to do that, we can use the information we found while exploring the Vitruvian Man, and what da Vinci wrote his notes. We saw that everybody tries to conform to this ratio of a body that is eight heads tall; and we also created an equation that represents that proportion, so let's begin by using this equation to find out how tall that person may have been. Let's look at Figure 4D to get a reminder of that equation.

b = body height

h = head length

$$\frac{b}{8} = h$$

Figure 4D

We see in the equation that if you divide any individual body height by eight; we can find the head length of that body, but we want to find the body height at the beginning of this model. In order for us to find this body height let's first use the one proportion of the human body with the least amount of variation. The one member of the body that could be used as our first unit that we can measure the standard measurement from would be the eye.

The proportion with the least amount of variation would be the eye proportion as it's compared to the head. The average diameter of the eye when we reach adulthood is about 25.4 mm; and with such a small variation in a measured size, we can then use the average of the eye to compare the rest of the body as an ideal model. In Figure 5D, we can see how this measurement will compare to the head; the eye is measured with the first whole number that begins within the set, at one inch. The eye, at one inch, is compared to the head; for every eight eyes is the measure for the beginning standard model for a head. Figure 5D gives an equation with one head; and it measures eight inches. So, if we use what we learned from Vitruvius; then we need to establish a set of comparable models that would be set to one unit of measure for every other model that has to be measured. Let's take a look at Figure 6D.

1 eye = 1 inch

8 eyes = 1 head

1 head = 8 inches

Figure 5D

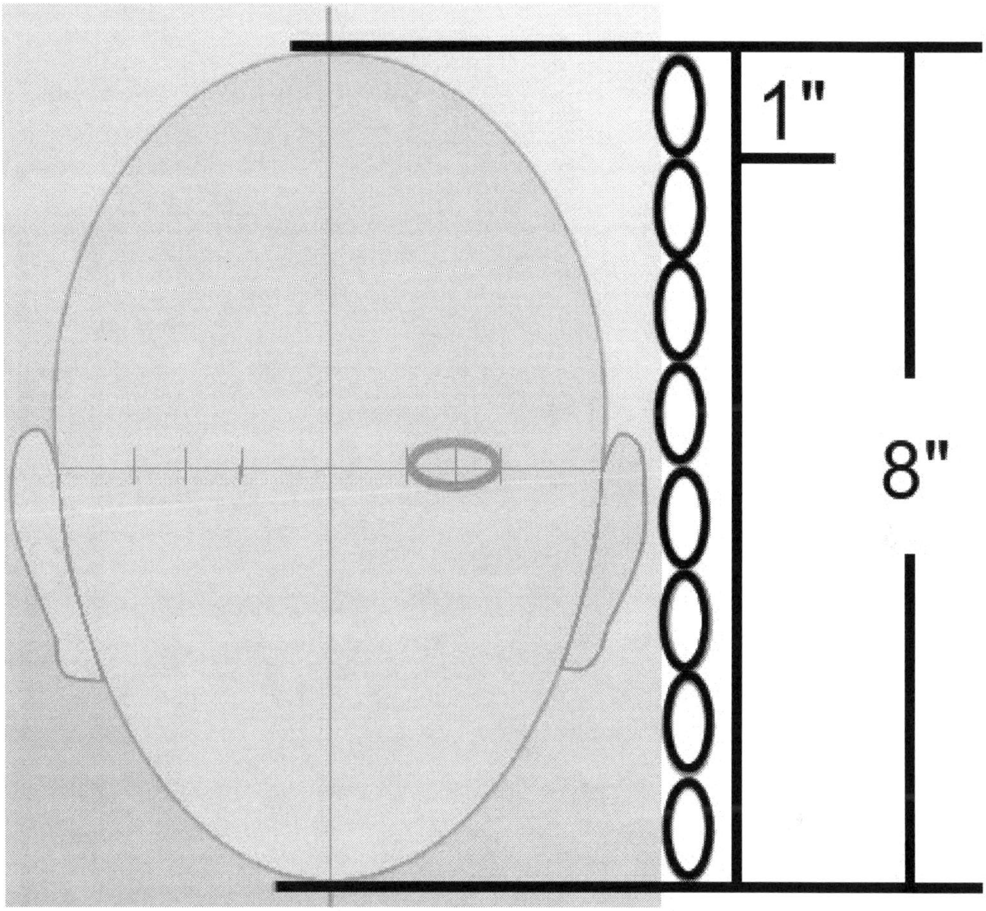

Figure 6D

In Figure 6D, we can see how this measurement would compare to the head; and we can also see the measurement of the head that would represent a head at the ideal model. This model is what we can assume to be within the equilibrium that everybody will try to attain as we reach adulthood. This will be the one general form of a head that we would have started at. This could have been the measurement of the head of what we would consider to be the very first human that walked upright.

1 head = 8 inches

8 heads = 1 body

1 body = 64 inches

Figure 7D

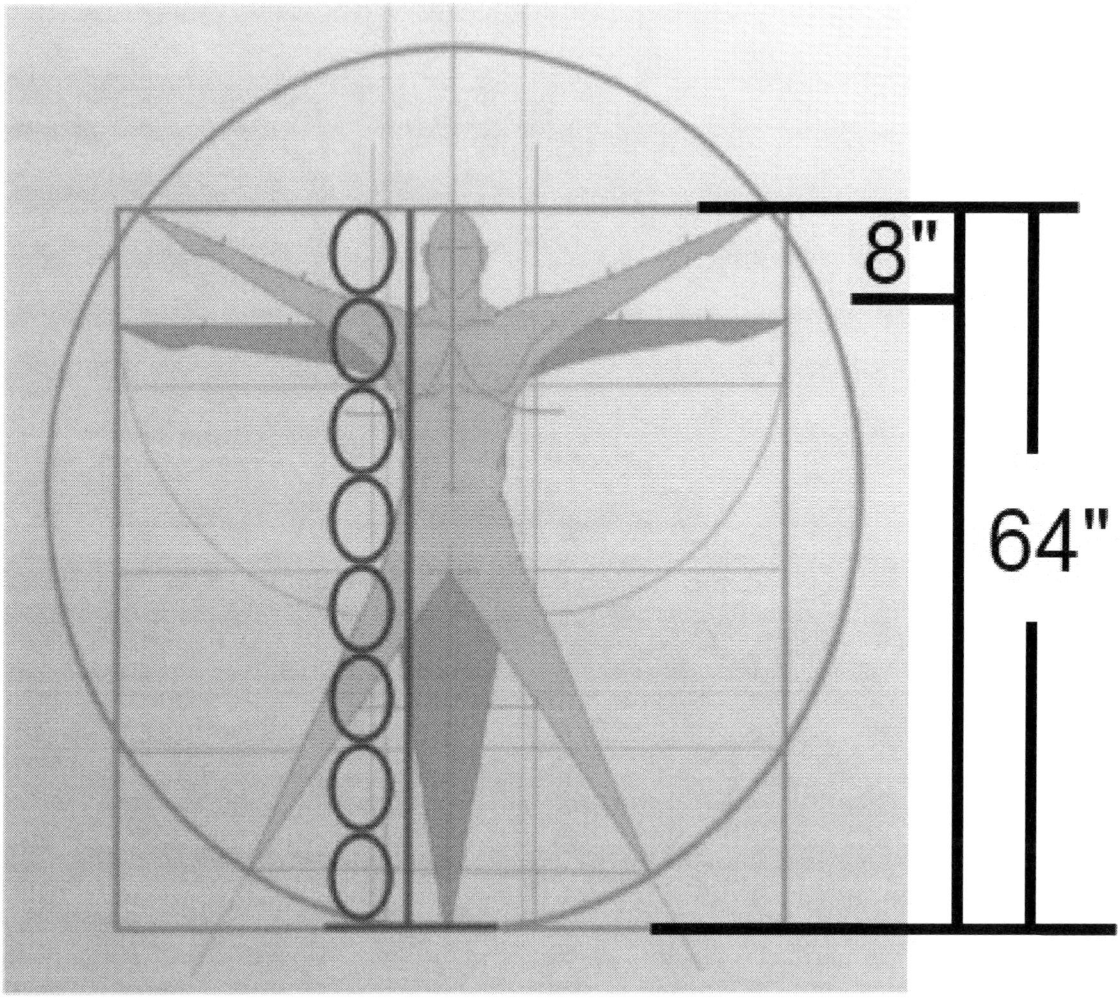

Figure 8D

In Figure 7D, we can find the one head measured as one unit to compare to the rest of the body; this would be the first whole unit within the model we have described in the book. One head would be measured as eight inches, eight heads will be the benchmark for one body unit, and then one body unit would be 64 inches tall, as seen in Figure 8D.

That would mean that this would be the first model of a human body as represented as compared to one unit per proportion of the three key features of a body that we have described throughout this book. This measurement doesn't represent the average human height of today; but it should give us an idea of what the earliest human might have looked like, compared to what modern humans look like.

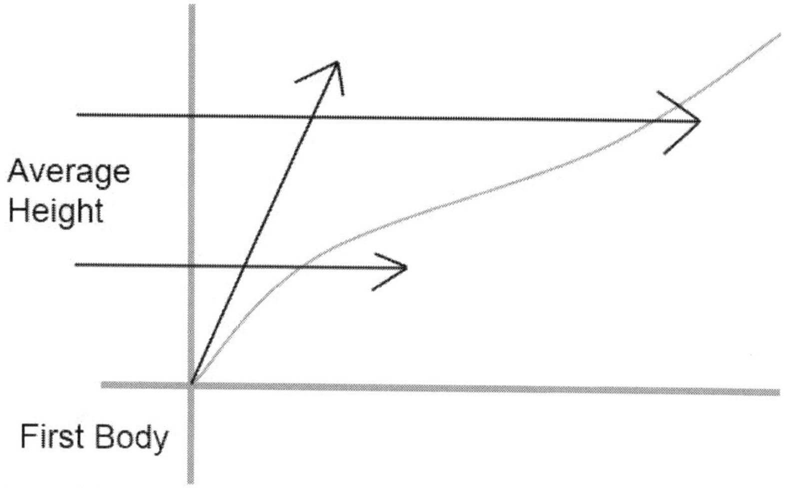

Figure 9D

The World English Dictionary defines mutation as "change in genetic material: a random change in a gene or chromosome resulting in a new trait or characteristic that can be inherited." [15] Since it is defined as a "change", then it would have to begin with a standard design to have changed from. We can see in Figure 9D; that as soon as the first body reached this model form, it would begin to mutate, or evolve, the average height over time would move away from this first model.

Our average body height at this time is around 5' 9" for an adult male; this average has changed so much over time, but we can still see this original model of a human body throughout our history. Studies have shown how our environment has lead to changes in our DNA over this time period; it has increased this change at some periods, and in other periods of history, we can see a decrease in this average. It all depends on how we have survived in our natural habitat that has made our body evolve away from that first model of what a human would look like.

If we used the same model that Vitruvius described; and we added what we learned in the book, then we could find a model that could be used to measure the rest of humanity. To begin with, we need to set our whole model of the human body to equal that one unit of measure for the body. This would be the start of a model; when it first reached the one to eight ratios, as compared to one whole unit of measure for the modern human body, and the measurements for that body. Let's take a close look at Figure 10D.

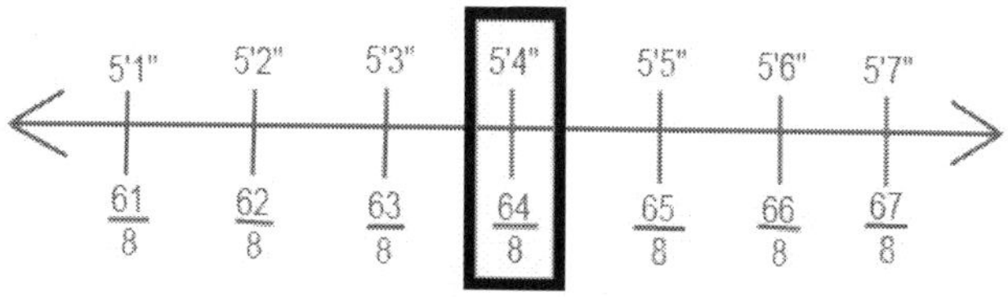

Figure 10D

For each different height, we only need to follow the scale up or down. This scale is infinite in both directions; as long as it remains within the same ratio. This scale is only for a body that has reached the 1 to 8 ratio. As we can see in Figure 10D, if a person is 65 inches tall, then they are also 5 feet 5 inches in height, and if divide 65 by 8, then we find the size of the head will be 8.125 inches in length.

This height would have been caused by either directly by design, or indirectly by a simple mutation. If it was indirectly caused by a mutation; then this mutation would have stuck, because it provided a better way to survive. If we take into account that at 64 inches; the body is at its ideal form and the mutation would have been strongest at this time, at this point in time the body would have been at its most ideal form of what a modern day human being would look like. It would have grown at the same rate as what an ideal form could have, and would have reached the basic model ratio at the same time. Once the growth of the body began to remain at this average; then the mutation would be stuck for good, and then as the population spread, we can see the average change in two directions, above the ideal form and below the ideal form. The average height may have changed over time, but the ratios of the members of the body still remain the same, therefore giving us two different rates to measure.

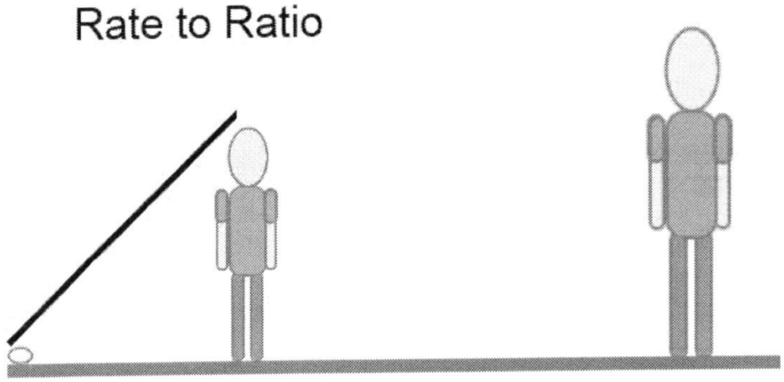

Figure 11D

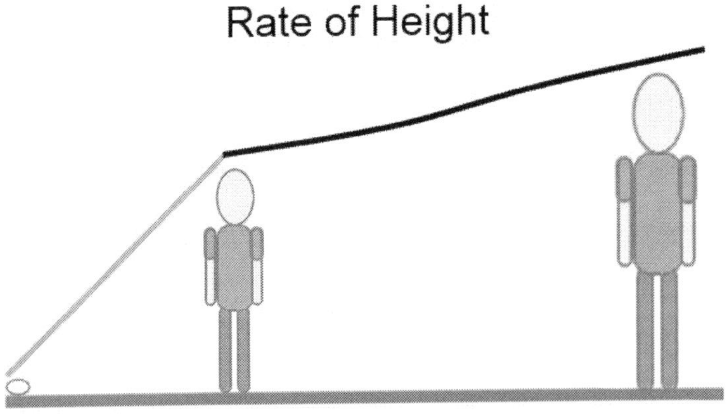

Figure 12D

At first each individual body will try to reach this ideal ratio; but then once it hits the ratio governed to it by the sum of the different mutations it may already have, as we can see in Figure 11D, it will stay at this ratio until death. The other rate; just after we reach this ratio, and the height of that whole system, now growing at the same rate, can be unique at different times in our life. The height of the body may change over time; the ratios of that body will remain the same.

There are two main versions of where we may have began; both with one Adam and one Eve. The biblical version of the story; tells us that we all come from the Adam and Eve, and that they were the first humans on the earth. This is what we learned in Sunday school; and if we assume that this is true, and then we should also assume that the basic form discussed throughout the book would be true. This design would have began with this Adam and Eve; and then passed down from there, evolving with each new generation. The body that we have found to be the basic model for the modern human body has the height of 64 inches, a head length of 8 inches, and an eye transverse length of 1 inch.

The second version of Adam and Eve is quite different, and a little harder to understand. The Mitochondrial Eve is so named because with new DNA research; they have found a way to use markers of when there was a significant mutation in the mitochondrial DNA passed down from mother to daughter, and they were able to trace it back as far as 200,000 years to a woman living in east Africa. They named her Mitochondrial Eve; because they can trace everyone's DNA back to her.

She was probably living with a whole tribe full of people, and there's no way to know for sure how many people were living at this time. The studies about this theory show that at some point after her time, the human species almost became extinct, and very few lines of human DNA survived. Those that did survive would have to have at least one line with Eve's DNA, and others may have survived also, but at some point all the others have disappeared from history. She would have been quite close to the basic model of what we have described.

Adam, in this same DNA search, is the one man we can trace our DNA back to, and the studies researching this could only trace it back to this point that was thousands of years later than Eve. That means only that they have still more research to link that line further back. That would also mean that he would have veered further away from the basic model than Eve.

If we were to assume that this design originated somewhere in the eastern part of Africa; then the oldest tribes there should also be the closest to the proportions of the original design for humanity.

Since the very first modern human, there has been no other perfect form of an ideal human body; only great, unexpected differences that have evolved to make our species so prolific, that it has spread all over the world, conquering almost any environment we can encounter.

Bibliography

1. Human Genome Project Information. U.S. Department of Energy Genome Programs. From the Genome to the Proteome. 26 March 2008. 6 Jan. 2011. http://www.ornl.gov/sci/techresources/Human Genome/project/info.shtml
2. WolfWikis. Group 6 HYALOS(hyaline cartilage). 31 Dec. 2010. http://wikis.lib.ncsu.edu/index.php/Group_6_HYALOS_(hyaline_cartilage)
3. Wikipedia. Vitruvius. 8 Nov. 2010. http://en.wikipedia.org/wiki/Vitruvius
4. Vitruvius. The Ten Books On Architecture. Trans. Morris Morgan, PH.D.,LL.D. 31 Dec.2006. 2 Feb. 2011. http://www.gutenburg.org/files/20239/20239-h/29239-h.htm
5. Leonardo da Vinci | Renaissance Man. Museum of Science, Boston. 6 Jan. 2011. http://www.mos.org/leonardo/bio.html
6. Wikipedia. Vitruvian Man. 30 Oct.2010. 3 Nov. 2010. http://en.wikipedia.org/wiki/Vitruvian Man
7. Suh, H. Anna,ed. "Leonardo's Notebooks" *Leonardo da Vinci.* New York, 2005.
8. Ask.com. Encyclopedia. Human Skull. 5 Nov. 2010 http://www.ask.com/wiki/Human skull
9. Song, Ha Tae, MD,et al. Relations between Age, Weight, Refractive Error and Eye Shape by Computerized Tomography in Children. National Center for Biotechnology Information. 31 July 2007. 27 Oct. 2010. http://www.ncbl.nlm.nih.gov/pmc/articles/PMC2629680/
10. Schudy, Fred, DDS MS. How Does the Human Head Grow? The Schudy Chronicles. 26 Oct. 2010. http://vsbw.com/~schudyf/art56.html
11. About.com. Pediatrics. Growth Chart: Boys Two to Twenty Years. Growth Chart: Girls Two to Twenty Years. 12 Jan. 2011. http://pediatrics.about.com/library/growth charts/nboystwo.htm http://pediatrics.about.com/library/growth charts/ngirlstwo.htm
12. Encarta. World English Dictionary. Proportion. 1998-2005 Microsoft Corporation.
13. Fledelius, Hans C. and Anders C. Christensen. Reappraisal of the Human Ocular Growth Curve in Fetal Life, Infancy, and Early Childhood. British Journal of Ophthalmology. 16 July 1996. 28 Oct. 2010. http://www.bjo.bmj.com
14. Webvision. Gross Anatomy of the Eye. 7 Feb. 2011. http://webvision.med.utah.edu/anatomy.html
15. Encarta. World English Dictionary. Mutation. 1998-2005 Microsoft Corporation.

Made in the USA
Monee, IL
08 November 2026

68156249R00063